Ventricular Assist Devices – Current Advances and Applications in Heart Failure

Edited by Enkhsaikhan Purevjav, Hugo Martinez, Jeffrey A. Towbin and Umar Boston

Published in London, United Kingdom

Ventricular Assist Devices - Current Advances and Applications in Heart Failure
http://dx.doi.org/10.5772/intechopen.102242
Edited by Enkhsaikhan Purevjav, Hugo Martinez, Jeffrey A. Towbin and Umar Boston

Contributors
Karen May-Newman, Vi Vu, Hugo R. Martinez, Neely R. Alberson, Ismael A. Salas De Armas, Jarot J. Guerra, David Garcia-Molinero, Rocio Toro, Michael A. Burke, Tamas Alexy, Karine Guerrier, Ahmad Sami Chaouki, Enkhsaikhan Purevjav, Buyan-Ochir Orgil, Jeffrey A. Towbin, Michael Sobieraj, Antonio Valone, Kulpreet Barn, Ricardo Chia, Brisha Bhikadiya, Marc O. Maybauer, Ammar Sharif, Joseph M. Brewer

First published in London, United Kingdom, 2023 by IntechOpen
IntechOpen is the global imprint of INTECHOPEN LIMITED, registered in England and Wales, registration number: 11086078, 5 Princes Gate Court, London, SW7 2QJ, United Kingdom

British Library Cataloguing-in-Publication Data
A catalogue record for this book is available from the British Library

Additional hard and PDF copies can be obtained from orders@intechopen.com

Ventricular Assist Devices - Current Advances and Applications in Heart Failure
Edited by Enkhsaikhan Purevjav, Hugo Martinez, Jeffrey A. Towbin and Umar Boston
p. cm.
Print ISBN 978-1-80356-452-4
Online ISBN 978-1-80356-453-1
eBook (PDF) ISBN 978-1-80356-454-8

Meet the editors

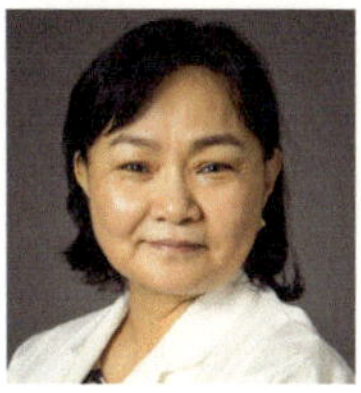

Dr. Purevjav is a Professor of Pediatrics at the University of Tennessee Health Science Center (UTHSC), USA. She is a fully trained pediatric cardiologist who earned her MD at the Leningrad Pediatric Medical Institute (LMPI), Russia, followed by an internship and residency in pediatrics at the Mongolian National Medical University and a clinical fellowship in Pediatric Cardiology and Electrophysiology at LPMI. After obtaining her Ph.D. in Medical Genetics and Molecular Biology at Shimane Medical University, Japan, Dr. Purevjav worked at Baylor College of Medicine and Texas Children's Hospital, USA, and Cincinnati Children's Hospital Medical Center, USA. As a professor at UTHSC, she continues to study the genetics, genomics, and systems genetics of heart diseases, specifically focusing on pediatric cardiomyopathies, arrhythmia disorders, and heart failure.

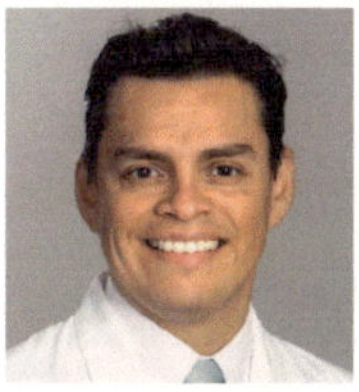

Dr. Hugo Martinez is an associate professor at the University of Tennessee Health Science Center (UTHSC), USA, and a certified pediatric cardiologist with experience in transplant cardiology, mechanical circulatory support, cardio-genetics, and cardio-oncology. At Le Bonheur Children's Hospital, he is the Director of the Cardiovascular Genetics clinic and the Medical Co-Director of the Heart Transplant Service Line. At St. Jude Children's Research Hospital, he serves as a consulting physician for the Cardio-Oncology Service. His work philosophy is to be creative and efficient in the management of children and young adults with cardiac dysfunction. His academic projects investigate novel therapeutic modalities for heart failure, the evaluation of cardio-genomic profiles, and the analysis of therapy-related cardiovascular dysfunction in children and young adults with cancer. Dr. Martinez has been published in textbooks and high-impact journals and has been invited to present at national and international conferences.

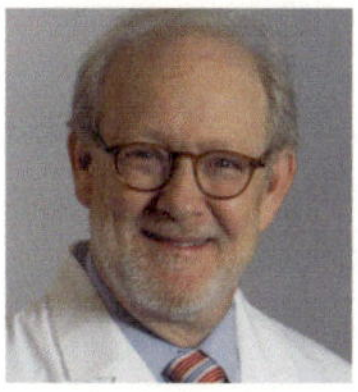

Jeffrey A. Towbin, MD, is executive co-director of the Heart Institute, chief of pediatric cardiology at Le Bonheur Children's Hospital and University of Tennessee Health Science Center (UTHSC), USA, and medical director of cardiomyopathy, heart failure, and transplant services. His interests include clinical, genetic, and mechanistic aspects of cardiomyopathies, arrhythmias, and sudden death with research focusing on gene identification and animal and cellular models. His 590 publications have generated new knowledge, allowing clarification of underlying pathophysiology, which guides targeted diagnostic and treatment options. Dr. Towbin is the recipient of the American College of Cardiology (ACC) Distinguished Scientist (Basic Science) Award (2007), Council on Cardiovascular Disease of the Young, American Heart Association (AHA) Meritorious Achievement Award (2010), AHA Basic Research Prize (2013), AHA Distinguished Scientist Award (2017), American Academy of Pediatrics Section on Cardiology and Cardiac Surgery Helen B. Taussig Founder's Award (2023), and the 2023 Heart Failure Society of America Pioneer Award.

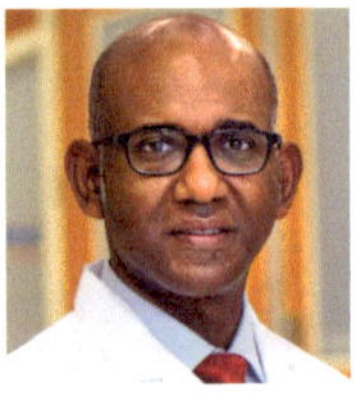

Umar Boston is a congenital heart surgeon who specializes in the surgical treatment of infants and children with heart failure. He is Professor of Surgery at the University of Tennessee Health Science Center (UTHSC), USA. He is a co-founder of the Pediatric Heart Transplant Program at Le Bonheur Children's Hospital, USA, where he currently serves as the surgical director of pediatric heart transplantation and ventricular assist device (VAD) service. He is nationally recognized for his innovative VAD strategies to bridge infants with failed single-ventricle palliation to heart transplantation. He is a member of numerous surgical societies including the International Society for Heart and Lung Transplantation, the Congenital Heart Surgeons' Society, and the and the Society of Thoracic Surgeons, to name a few.

Contents

Preface **IX**

Section 1
History of Mechanical Circulatory Support in Heart Failure **1**

Chapter 1 **3**
A Historical Review of Mechanical Circulatory Support
by Hugo Martinez, Neely R. Alberson, Jarot J. Guerra and Ismael A. Salas De Armas

Section 2
Cardiac Remodeling Related to Mechanical Circulatory Support **21**

Chapter 2 **23**
Myocardial Remodeling with Ventricular Assist Devices
by Buyan-Ochir Orgil, Neely R. Alberson, Jeffrey A. Towbin and Enkhsaikhan Purevjav

Section 3
Arrhythmia Management during Mechanical Circulatory Support **49**

Chapter 3 **51**
Arrhythmia Management in Pediatric Patients with Ventricular Assist Devices
by Karine Guerrier and Ahmad Sami Chaouki

Chapter 4 **65**
Implantable Cardioverter-Defibrillator Use in Patients with Left Ventricular Assist Devices
by David Garcia-Molinero and Rocio Toro

Section 4
Management of Complications during Mechanical Circulatory Support **81**

Chapter 5 **83**
Recurrent Heart Failure after Left Ventricular Assist Device Placement
by Tamas Alexy and Michael A. Burke

Chapter 6 **113**
Aortic Insufficiency in LVAD Patients
by Vi Vu and Karen May-Newman

Chapter 7 **133**
Perspective Chapter: The ProtekDuo® Cannula for Acute Mechanical Circulatory Support
by Joseph M. Brewer, Ammar Sharif and Marc O. Maybauer

Section 5
Delivery of Mechanical Circulatory Support Care to Remote Communities **155**

Chapter 8 **157**
Perspective Chapter: Delivering LVAD Care to the Local Community
by Michael Sobieraj, Antonio Valone, Brisha Bhikadiya, Ricardo Chia and Kulpreet Barn

Preface

Heart failure is a condition of diminished blood pumping by the heart that causes poor delivery of oxygen and nutrients to vital organs and the rest of the body. Heart failure is a devastating disease with high mortality. Its incidence is expected to rise by nearly 30% from the current 6.2 million affected people to almost 8 million by 2030 in the United States alone. This book covers broad but important aspects of mechanical circulatory support (MCS) with ventricular assist devices (VAD) that support patients with advanced and end-stage heart failure.

This book, a collection of review papers from experienced and knowledgeable physicians and scientists, provides an overview of the history of MCS devices, including their development, optimization, and application to the treatment and management of heart failure. The authors emphasize the importance of diagnosis and treatment strategies for common risks and complications that patients encounter during MSC, such as arrhythmias, recurrent heart failure, aortic insufficiency, and acute hypertension. These complications increase morbidity and mortality in patients with VAD. The chapter that describes the use of implanted cardioverter defibrillators in various clinical situations related to VAD is a valuable resource for medical personnel in preventing sudden death and complications during MCS therapy. The book also includes comprehensive reviews of basic, translational, and human research focusing on cardiac remodeling and the underlying molecular, cellular, and circulatory mechanisms that evolve in response to ventricular unloading with MCS devices. A chapter on assessment and management for better delivery of MCS care to local communities, particularly those patients who live in rural and remote areas, adds valuable information that can be adopted in many hospitals to improve the benefits and quality of VAD care.

The editors are delighted to present *Ventricular Assist Devices – Advances and Applications in Heart Failure* for a broad audience of physicians, surgeons, and scientists who work to save the lives of patients with heart failure.

Enkhsaikhan Purevjav, MD, Ph.D., FAHA
The Heart Institute,
The University of Tennessee Health Science Center,
Memphis, Tennessee, USA

Children's Foundation Research Institute,
Le Bonheur Children's Hospital,
Memphis, Tennessee, USA

Hugo Martinez, MD
Pediatric Cardiology and Genetics,
The University of Tennessee Health Science Center,
Memphis, Tennessee, USA

The Heart Institute,
Le Bonheur Children's Hospital,
Memphis, Tennessee, USA

Jeffrey A. Towbin
The Heart Institute,
The University of Tennessee Health Science Center,
Memphis, Tennessee, USA

Children's Foundation Research Institute,
Le Bonheur Children's Hospital,
Memphis, Tennessee, USA

Pediatric Cardiology,
St. Jude Children's Research Hospital,
Memphis, Tennessee, USA

Umar Boston, MD
Pediatric Cardiology,
The University of Tennessee Health Science Center,
Memphis, Tennessee, USA

The Heart Institute,
Le Bonheur Children's Hospital,
Memphis, Tennessee, USA

Section 1

History of Mechanical Circulatory Support in Heart Failure

Chapter 1

A Historical Review of Mechanical Circulatory Support

Hugo Martinez, Neely R. Alberson, Jarot J. Guerra and Ismael A. Salas De Armas

Abstract

Meaningful and contemporary data regarding the clinical use of mechanical circulatory support (MCS) is founded on the work conducted in the 1950s when a "heart-lung" machine was incorporated to provide support during surgical interventions. Following this milestone, the need to support artificial circulation in patients with heart failure initiated an investigational and legislative collaboration to implement the mission-oriented Artificial Heart Program in the United States during the 1960s. In the subsequent decades, technological discoveries have integrated a series of mechanical systems employed as therapeutic options for short- and long-term artificial circulation in children and adults with advanced heart failure. Since their clinical application, MCS devices have been employed as a bridge to transplantation in over 4000 patients globally. In recent years, the adverse effects and economic burden of MCS have been counterbalanced by the harmonization of therapeutic protocols, the inclusion of multidisciplinary insight, and the allowance of families and patients to participate in shared decision making to address candidacy. In this chapter, we provide a review of the historical aspects of MCS, a therapeutic option for overcoming complexities encountered in reestablishing adequate hemodynamic states and providing a reasonable quality of life.

Keywords: mechanical circulatory support, heart failure, historical aspects, left ventricular assist device, destination therapy

1. Introduction

Heart failure (HF) affects approximately 6 million adults in the United States (US) and is projected to affect over 8 million persons over the age of 18 years by the year 2030 [1]. Of these, it is estimated that the prevalence of advanced heart failure (American College of Cardiology/American Heart Association Stage D) ranges between 250,000 and 300,000 individuals. Between 1988 and 2021, over 83,000 heart transplants were performed in the US. Among those patients, a ventricular assist device (VAD) was used in over 20,000 or approximately 25% of transplantations [2]. Pediatric patients (≤17 years old) comprised 31% of total transplantations, and approximately 9% of children required a VAD as a bridge to transplantation (BTT) [2].

A description of noteworthy milestones in the history of cardiac surgery and mechanical support must include the meaningful advances led by Dr. John H. Gibbon in the 1950s. These advances laid the foundation for the use of cardiopulmonary bypass (CPB) and circulatory assist devices to support patients with perioperative complications and prolonged hemodynamic recovery [3, 4]. Since the early days of mechanical circulatory support (MCS), VADs have become a standardized alternative strategy to bridge to hemodynamic recovery, destination therapy, a bridge during decision-making for the next steps in management, or as a BTT [5].

The first clinical use of a LVAD was reported by Liotta *et al.* in 1963, in a patient with cardiac arrest the morning after aortic valve replacement. The intrathoracic pump was still functioning 4 days postoperatively when the patient died due to brain damage, a complication of cardiac arrest they experienced prior to LVAD implantation [6]. In 1964, The National Institutes of Health (NIH) became actively involved in the development of mechanical assist devices with the inception of the Artificial Heart Program [7]. By 1966, the first successful pneumatically driven paracorporeal left ventricular assist device (LVAD) was employed by DeBakey et al. to support a patient following cardiac surgery. The first human heart transplant was performed by Dr. Christiaan Barnard in 1967, and shortly afterward the use of artificial ventricle technology was initiated as a bridge to support patients until a donor heart could be found [8–10]. Concurrently, the idea of replacing the entire organ using an "artificial pump" came to clinical practice in 1969 by Cooley *et al.* who reported the first use of a total artificial heart (TAH) as a BTT. However, this device was only able to be retained for a few days due to adverse events such as infection, thrombosis, and hemolysis [11].

The establishment of the National Heart, Lung, and Blood Institute (NHLBI) by the NIH in the 1970s promoted the development of implantable devices intending to provide longer mechanical support [7]. In 1978, the first LVAD was used by Norman et al. for nearly 6 days as a BTT [12]. The first TAH intended for permanent support was implanted in 1984 by DeVries et al. with the patient being supported for 112 days before succumbing to sepsis [13].

The first successful BTT case using a VAD was reported by Portner *et al.* in 1984 using the Novacor (Baxter Healthcare Corporation, Oakland, CA) implantable electrical LVAD in a patient with ischemic end-stage heart disease [14]. By the mid-1990s, the FDA approved multiple pulsatile devices allowing patients to recover from hemodynamic compromise [15] (**Figure 1**). Subsequently, in the Randomized Evaluation of Mechanical Assistance for the Treatment of Congestive Heart Failure (REMATCH) trial, a new indication for mechanical support was explored and the trial revealed

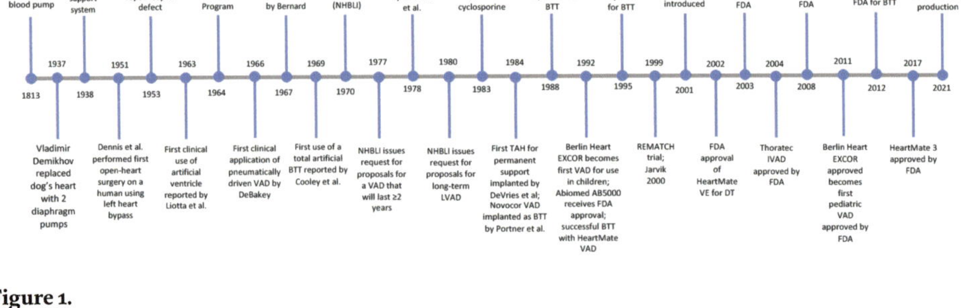

Figure 1.
Important milestones in the history of mechanical circulatory support.

that patients supported by a LVAD exhibited an 81% improvement in 2-year survival compared to medical therapy in patients with advanced heart failure who were not candidates for heart transplantation [5, 16]. The results of this trial led to the approval of the HeartMate VE LVAD device for destination therapy in 2003.

As the prevalence of advanced heart failure increased over the past decades, utilization of LVADs became essential to improve pre-transplant illnesses, improve quality of life, and enhance survivorship—a phenomenon primarily driven by advances in device design, patient characteristics, implantation techniques, and long-term management of adverse effects [17, 18].

2. Ventricular assist devices

2.1 First generation

The earliest VADs incorporated a diaphragm and unidirectional artificial valves to replicate the pulsatile cardiac cycle with a diastolic filling time and a systolic emptying of the devices, mimicking that of the native heart [19]. These devices are pumps designed to mechanically assist a failing Left Ventricle (LV) by removing blood from the LV and returning it into the circulatory system *via* the aorta. While LV dysfunction is more common, VADs can also be used to treat right ventricular failure or both. These first-generation VADs were either pneumatically or electrically driven, included the Thoratec HeartMate IP ("Implantable Pneumatic"), VE ("Vented Electric"), XVE ("Extended Vented Electric") (Abbott Laboratories, formerly Thoratec, Pleasanton, CA), and the Berlin Heart EXCOR (Berlin Heart, Berlin, Germany) [1]. These early devices were used to support patients as a BTT and could be used as left-, right-, and biventricular devices (LVAD, RVAD, and BiVAD). The first-generation devices introduced electromechanical actuation, which allowed some to be powered by a battery worn on the waist, affording better mobility, and allowing patients to be discharged from the hospital waiting for a new heart [20]. Anecdotally, these first devices had several disadvantages including large size, noise emission, infectious diseases, malfunctioning, mechanical tears, or valve degradation.

First-generation LVADs were known as volume displacement pumps and generated flow *via* a pulse generator [15, 21]. The goal of the first-generation LVADs was to provide long-term circulatory support, such that these devices could be used as a bridge to transplant [20, 22].

The HeartMate systems were housed within a titanium shell and situated beneath the patient's diaphragm on the left side. Within the housing, a polyurethane diaphragm divided the blood-contacting chamber and the chamber housing the motor. A sintered titanium microsphere layer was applied to the titanium blood-contacting surfaces of the pump and a fibrillar texture was on the polyurethane diaphragm. These surface modifications allowed circulating cells to adhere and form an intima-like tissue layer [20, 22]. The HeartMate IP (Abbott Laboratories, formerly Thoratec, Pleasanton, CA, USA) was the first LVAD to receive FDA approval for use in patients as a BTT in 1994. Clinical trials of the HeartMate VE began in 1992. Following the positive outcomes from the REMATCH trial, the HeartMate VE was approved by the FDA as destination therapy in 2003. This VAD was later updated to the HeartMate XVE device and served as the device to which the next generation of LVAD was compared. The Heartmate VE and XVE systems were driven by an electric motor. The REMATCH results propelled widespread use of LVADs in the clinical setting and led to FDA approval of the HeartMate VE (HeartMate I) and the inclusion of other first-generation LVADs such as the Thoratec Implantable VAD (IVAD), an intracorporeal device, as well as the Thoratec PVAD, a paracorporeal device. Both devices provide the option of being used as left, right, or biventricular support and are both approved for use as BTTs. They were pulsatile flow devices comprising a 65-mL blood chamber with unidirectional flow achieved by tilting disk mechanical valves [23].

The Novacor LVAS (formerly WorldHeart, Oakland, CA, and acquired by HeartWare International, Inc., Framingham, MA) features an implanted pump/drive unit and an external control console. The pump consisted of a polyurethane sac bonded to dual pusher plates contained in a housing that included valve fittings. This device became available in 1984, initially as a console-based unit, but a wearable configuration became available in 1993. This unit was initially intended for destination therapy (DT) in the treatment of individuals with end-stage heart failure, but it was eventually used as a BTT [24]. The first clinical implant for a bridge to transplantation reportedly occurred in 1984 by Portner et al. [25]. Complications associated with the device included cerebral vascular accidents, bleeding, and infection. This device was discontinued by the manufacturer in 2008 with a greater focus on newer-generation VADs.

The Arrow LionHeart LVAD 2000 (Arrow International Inc., Reading, PA) was an implantable pulsatile VAD, designed for use for DT in patients with end-stage heart failure. The system had no percutaneous lines or connections and consisted of a titanium blood pump with inflow and outflow assemblies, a motor, a compliance chamber, and a transcutaneous energy transmission system [26]. The Clinical Utility Baseline Study was performed to establish whether the transcutaneous energy transmission system resulted in fewer infections than the observed during the REMATCH trial and concluded that Lionheart recipients exhibited less sepsis and device-related infection than the REMATCH trial group. The device, however, was discontinued in 2005.

The Berlin Heart EXCOR VAD was developed in Berlin, Germany, by Berlin Heart and is a pneumatically driven paracorporeal support device that can be used to provide left, right, or biventricular support. Its size ranges from pediatric to adult sizes. The device was first used as a BTT in 1988 [27, 28]. In 1992, the Berlin Heart became the first commercially available pulsatile assist device for children. This device received the CE mark in Europe in 2000 but was granted FDA approval for pediatric use only in the USA in 2011. This device is specifically designed for infants and children with stroke volumes of 10, 25, and 30 mL [29]. It is a pneumatic, compressor-operated diaphragm pump with polyurethane valves. Larger pumps (50, 60, and 80 mL) are equipped with mechanical valves.

BiVADs may be useful in patients with total heart failure and support both sides of the heart by balancing left and right pump flows. First-generation BiVADs included Abiomed BVS5000 and AB5000 (AbioMed Inc., Danvers, MA, USA), Thoratec PVAD and IVAD (Thoratec), Berlin Heart EXCOR (Berlin Heart, Berlin, Germany), and Medos HIA-VAD (MEDOS Medizintechnic GmbH, Stolberg, Germany) [2].

The Abiomed BVS5000 (AbioMed) was clinically introduced in 1987 and approved for use by the FDA in 1992. The device is an extracorporeal, dual-chambered BiVAD. The advantages of this device include simplicity and low cost, making it one of the most frequently used BiVADs worldwide [30]. The BVS5000 has two separate pumping and filling bladders driven by a pulsatile drive console. The device has demonstrated reasonable success in bridging patients to recovery from cardiogenic shock; however, issues with portability and thrombus incidence present limitations should long-term VAD support be required [31]. The Abiomed AB5000 (AbioMed) gained FDA approval in 2003 and is very similar to the BVS5000, as it is a pneumatically driven volume displacement pump. Unlike the BVS5000, its paracorporeal location means that this device can be used as a VAD treatment or as a replacement, allowing the patient greater mobility [32].

The Thoratec PVAD (Thoratec) was approved by the FDA in 1995 for BTT and in 1998 for postcardiotomy support. It is a pneumatically driven paracorporeal VAD suited for left, right, or biventricular assistance, as well as use as a total artificial heart. The Thoratec IVAD (Thoratec) was approved by the FDA in 2004 to support systemic and/or pulmonary circulations in left, right, or biventricular assist configuration. This device is intracorporeal, pneumatically actuated, and pulsatile, operating in a full-to-empty mode utilizing optical infrared sensors to detect the end-systolic and diastolic position of the membrane providing an adequate balance of blood flow [33].

The Medos HIA-VAD is a paracorporeal device with transparent pump chamber sizes to be used in adult, infant, and pediatric cases. Development was initiated in 1982 at Helmholtz Institute for Biomedical Engineering in Aachen, Germany, and was acquired by Medos Medizintechnik GmbH in 1990. It has been used since 1994 and received the CE trademark in Europe in 1997. The system can work either at a fixed rate or with an electrocardiogram trigger and is pneumatically actuated, providing left, right, or biventricular support [15, 19].

The NIPRO-VAD (National Cardiovascular Center/Toyobo ventricular assist system) is an extracorporeal pneumatically driven diaphragm pump. It was reportedly first implanted in 1982 at the Saitama University Medical School and the Osaka University Hospital. While the device has been used long term, up to 1264 days, patients supported by this system have limited mobility and therefore the device has been exchanged for second- and third-generation devices [22].

The Zeon VAD is a pneumatically driven extracorporeal pump, first implanted in 1980. The pump was used for left, right, and biventricular support as BTT in Japan. The pump was discontinued in 2005 [22].

2.2 Second generation

Since first-generation pumps were limited by their large size, high noise emissions, decreased patient mobility, and durability issues, research to develop smaller, more reliable devices was initiated [15]. Some of the features that characterize the second-generation LVADs from the first are that they are continuous, rather than pulsatile pumps, and that they produce axial blood motion using a rotor [34]. The second- and third-generation VADs replace or support only the ventricular function. There is no direct attempt made to imitate the modality of the native, ventricular function [20, 34].

The first reported device that falls in the second-generation category is the Biomedicus Bio-Pump (Medtronic Inc., Eden Praire, MN, USA). It has been used since the mid-1980s. Is a centrifugal pump that provides extracorporeal left and/or right ventricular assistance for short-term bridge-to-bridge, bridge-to-recovery, and bridge-to-transplant support [34, 35].

The HemoPump was the first implantable rotary blood pump with an extracorporeal drive. It required continuous infusion of a purge fluid. It was only used within clinical trials in the USA and the first in man use was in 1988, marking the beginning of the era of implantable, less invasive, rotary ventricular assist devices [36].

A few years later in Europe, in 1999, the ROTAFLOW (Maquet, Hirrlingen, Germany) was approved for pulmonary and/or ventricular support, including cardiopulmonary bypass, or used in the framework of extracorporeal membrane oxygenation (ECMO) procedures [34].

The first clinical use in a human of the DeBakey VAD, which later evolved to the HeartAssist 5, was in November 1998, and this marks the beginning of a new era of long-term second-generation LVADs. The VAD itself consists of a miniaturized axial flow pump system, an external controller system, and a clinical data acquisition system [37, 38]. This is the only rotary LVAD where the flow is measured directly at the outflow prosthesis with an ultrasonic transducer, thereby producing reliable system monitoring [38].

After a decade of pioneering work achieved with the HemoPump, the Impella product family evolved into a platform technology. In 1999, the Impella device was approved for use in Europe. The Impella RP (AbioMed Inc., Danvers, MA, USA) is a minimally invasive temporary microaxial pump for the percutaneous treatment of RV failure in pediatric or adult patients for up to 14 days. The device is exclusively inserted percutaneously through the femoral vein and advanced in an antegrade fashion across the pulmonary valve into the pulmonary artery under fluoroscopy. The pump aspirates blood from the inferior vena cava and ejects it into the pulmonary artery. This action provides forward flow in the pulmonary circulation and unloading of the RV [39]. The Impella 2.5, CP, 5.0, 5.5, and LD have also been designed and approved for use in High-Risk Percutaneous Coronary Interventions (HRPCI) and cardiogenic shock [34].

The Impella 2.5 and CP are percutaneous microaxial circulatory support pumps. The Impella 2.5 can deliver up to 2.5 l/min of systemic flow augmentation by pumping directly from the left ventricle into the ascending aorta [40]. The Impella CP can deliver flows up to 3.7 l/min. The Impella 2.5 and CP are used for HRPCI. The Impella 2.5 showed better results in patients undergoing HRPCI than the intra-aortic balloon pump [41]. In addition, the Impella CP due to easy placement access through the femoral artery, can be used in cases of acute decompensated heart failure or worsening cardiogenic shock driven by the left ventricle.

The Impella 5.0 and 5.5 are larger microaxial pumps implanted through a conduit sutured to the axillary artery [42] or directly sutured to the aorta through a graft either through a full sternotomy or through partial upper one in cases of small axillary artery [43] and can provide flows, 5.0 and 5.5 l/min, respectively, like that of durable LVADs [44]. They also promote patient mobilization and therefore give patients the ability to participate in physical therapy. They can also be used when other smaller microaxial pumps result in refractory hemolysis, resulting in better outcomes [45]. The Impella 5.5 can be used in cardiogenic shock as a bridge to recovery, a bridge to transplant, a bridge to a decision, or a durable LVAD [46].

The Jarvik 2000 FlowMaker (Jarvik Heart, Inc., New York, NY) is an axial flow LVAD that has been used in patients since the year 2000 as a bridge to recovery (BTR), BTT, and DT. This device uses alternative outflow connections and can also be used to support right ventricular function in humans. The pump is equipped with five speeds that can be manually set [47]. It is one of the smallest clinically available LVADs as well as having the longest period of left ventricular support with 9.5 years of uninterrupted support [16].

In 2001, Thoratec introduced the most successful LVAD, with respect to implantation numbers and studies, the HeartMate II VAD which was smaller and lighter than the original HeartMate XVE [3] (**Figure 2**). The development was initiated in

1991 with research collaboration between the McGowan Center of the University of Pittsburgh and Nimbus Company [20, 34]. It was approved for use in 2005 in Europe and the USA, the FDA approved it as a BTT device in 2008 and as a DT device in 2010. It is an axial-flow device composed of a blood pump, percutaneous lead, an external power source, and a system driver. The pump rotor and blood tube are made of smooth titanium, while the stators, inlet and outlet elbows, and intraventricular cannula are textured with titanium microsphere coatings. This design reduced prothrombotic sites and minimized wear and tear associated with multiple moving parts. Surfaces contacted by blood were designed with a textured titanium lining as an antithrombotic measure. Initially, the pump was placed in the intra-abdominal position but was then switched to a preperitoneal position where the body of the pump can then be easily accessed for pump exchange through a left subcostal approach [48]. From 2009 to 2017, the HeartMate 2 was the main LVAD being implanted worldwide. Although the improvement of survival over time has led to widespread adoption of this therapy, adverse events persist including, infection, bleeding, and pump thrombosis [49]. The rate of pump thrombosis has been reported as high as 10% after the first-year post-implantation, with a rate of 13% of pump exchange secondary to pump thrombosis [50]. One cause of driveline failure in the HeartMate II is damage to the wiring insulation of the percutaneous lead resulting in an electrical short to ground, referred to as a short-to-shield (STS). The percutaneous lead has six electrical wires attached to six motor stators to power a three-phase pump. There are three stranded primary wires and three backup wires for each of the phases. An STS occurs when there is an inappropriate electrical connection between one of the stranded wires and the shield, disrupting the normal flow of power [51]. A phase-to-phase short occurs when there is a loss of insulation between the three redundant motor coils (i.e., phases) of the driveline. When present, phase-to-phase short is particularly troublesome in that pump stoppages are likely and unpredictable. The manufacturer, therefore, recommended against controller exchange due to concern over the possibility that the pump would not restart, and instead recommended driveline repair, followed by surgical pump exchange should the problem persist [52]. Currently, there are still thousands of patients supported with the HeartMate 2 pump, **Figure 2**.

The CircuLite Synergy Micro-Pump, unlike the HemoPump and the Impella, was approved as a long-term LVAD and was implanted for the first time in a human in 2007. This pump was mainly used as a partial support device and sits in a pacemaker-like pocket [34].

The EVAHEART is the only implantable, centrifugal second-generation LVAD. The first-in-human use was in 2005 and was approved in Japan in 2010. It requires continuous insertion of cool seal fluid (purified water) [34].

The Heartmate X was announced in 2012 as an axial LVAD and leverages HeartMate 2 core bearing technology and is still under development in the animal stage [34]. It is a smaller pump and potentially allows for a less invasive implantation technique and could be used for smaller patients [53].

The Thoratec PHP was approved in Europe in 2015, which was the last approval of the second-generation LVADs, consisting of a shaft-driven axial pump with a foldable impeller. The device is inserted through the femoral artery and advanced to the aortic valve.

The MERA HCF-MP23 (Senki Medical Instrument Manufacturing Co. Ltd., Tokyo, Japan) is a centrifugal pump used for short-term extracorporeal circulatory support. The use is aimed at open heart surgery circulatory support and for bridge-to-decision

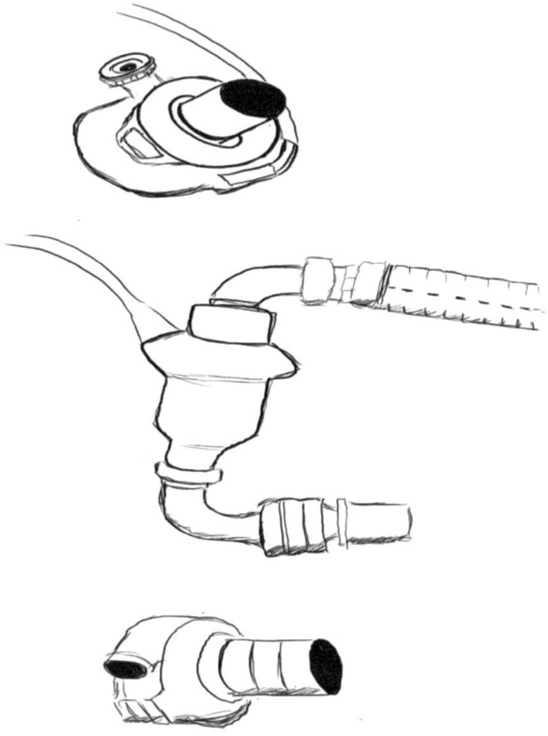

Figure 2.
Schematic representation of the HeartMate II (Abbott Laboratories, Abbott Park, IL). A successful continuous-flow pump with axial design.

use for up to 4 weeks. However, it was successfully used as an RVAD in a patient with right heart failure post-LVAD implantation for up to 17 weeks [54].

2.3 Third generation

Third-generation LVADs are continuous-flow centrifugal pumps designed with magnetic and/or hydrodynamic levitation of the impeller with non-contact bearings and outflow directed perpendicular to the axis of rotation [15, 19, 20, 55]. Fully magnetically levitated implantable blood pumps were proposed in patients by Olsen and Bramm in 1986 and Moise in 1987 [55]. Currently, continuous flow LVADs (CF-LVADs) are used in 99% of patients requiring an LVAD [30]. The development of third-generation devices aimed to improve durability and hemocompatibility. The two main LVADs discussed in this chapter are HeartMate III and HeartWare. Other examples include the TandemHeart (CardiacAssist Inc., Pittsburgh, PA, USA), Levacor (World Heart Inc., Salt Lake City, UT), and the DuraHeart (Teruma Heart, Inc., Ann Arbor, MI).

The HeartWare HVAD (Medtronic Inc., FL, USA) was approved by the FDA for BTT in 2012 and its implantation is completely intrapericardial; a smaller pump size eliminates the need for an abdominal pocket [30, 55]. From 2012 to 2017 was the pump of choice as BTT and for an additional year was the pump most commonly implanted as destination therapy. This device has magnetic and hydrodynamic levitation of the internal rotor and is connected directly to the heart at the base of the left ventricle. This device had the advantage that could be implanted without cardiopulmonary bypass easily due to the design of the coring knife [56]. The FDA recalled this device and Medtronic halted distribution and sale in June 2021 due to increased risk of neurological events and mortality associated with the internal pump, and the ability to restart if the internal pump stops [57].

The HeartMate III (Abbott Laboratories, formerly Thoratec Corporation, Pleasanton, CA, USA) was initially approved by the FDA for adults awaiting a heart transplant in 2017 and approved for long-term use in 2018. Its initial development started in 1998, using the same technology as the CentriMag, but modified to be fully implantable [55]. The first in human use was in June 2014. This device is implanted directly into the left ventricle and is fully magnetically levitated. It is designed to pass an inflow cannula through the apex of the heart and is directed toward the mitral valve to optimally drain blood from the left ventricle through the outflow graft and into the systemic circulation. The implications of this technology are substantial. Data from the MOMENTUM three randomized trial and subsequent publications (including the 5-year follow-up) have demonstrated the superiority of the centrifugal-flow LVAD to the HeartMate II with respect to survival to transplant, recovery, or LVAD support free of debilitating stroke or reoperation [58]. The superior performance of the HM3 at 6 months was due to 0% of the HM3 patients experiencing pump thrombosis, whereas 10.1% of patients with HM2 experienced pump thrombosis. Significant differences were not appreciated when comparing HM3 and HM2 with respect to bleeding, sepsis, driveline infection, right heart failure, arrhythmia, respiratory failure, renal dysfunction, hepatic dysfunction, or hemolysis not associated with pump thrombosis.

The HeartMate 6, an off-label use of two HeartMate 3 devices for biventricular support as a total artificial heart, has been reported in a patient as a successful bridge to transplant [59].

The Abbott CentriMag was the first available third-generation blood pump that was fully magnetically levitated. Originally developed and commercialized by Levitronix in 1995, the medical arm of Levitronix was then acquired by Thoratec in 2011 and Thoratec was later acquired by Abbott in January 2017 [55]. It is an extracorporeal centrifugal pump and is approved for use as an RVAD for up to 30 days in patients with cardiogenic shock. The magnetic levitation and motor principles are identical to those of the HeartMate 3, described above. Cannulation configuration differs depending on the support needed, i.e., LVAD, RVAD, or BiVAD. The CentriMag can also be used as a pump in the ECMO circuit [55].

In the US, it is approved for 6-hour acute extracorporeal circulatory support during cardiac surgery or humanitarian use device for RVAD support in cardiogenic shock as a result of right-sided heart failure. It is the surgical temporary ventricular assist device of choice. In Europe, it is approved for 30 days of extracorporeal VAD support [55].

The Levacor LVAD (WorldHeart has ceased trading) development was originally started by Medquest in 1996 and then was later acquired by WorldHeart. The first in human use was in March 2006. It is a radial flow pump employing a hybrid active and passive bearing to suspend a centrifugal impeller. In 2011, World Heart discontinued efforts to commercialize this device as a result of large device size and technical issues [60].

The Terumo DuraHeart LVAD (Terumo Corporation, Tokyo, Japan) was developed in 1991 with its first human use in January 2014. It is an implantable radial flow pump incorporating an axial magnetic bearing providing long-term left ventricular assistance with a contact-free impeller suspension system. The US SUSTAIN trial (A Study Evaluating Safety and Effectiveness of the DuraHeart Left Ventricular Assist System in Bridge to Transplant Patients) began in 2008 but was prematurely terminated in December 2011, due to slow recruitment based on the size of the device and the difficult configuration of the inflow cannula [61].

The HeartWare MVAD (Medtronic Inc., FL, USA) is a miniaturized implantable VAD that uses a passive maglev and hydrodynamic bearing system to levitate the rotor once it is rotating. It was developed in 2004 with the first in human use in July 2015. Its clinical trial was suspended 2 months later and has not been restarted [55].

The TandemHeart (CardiacAssist Inc., Pittsburgh, PA, USA) uses a paracorporeal, continuous flow, centrifugal pump originally developed for left atrial-to-femoral artery bypass to provide hemodynamic support during high-risk coronary interventions and post-cardiotomy cardiac failure. It was first used in a human in the year 2000 The use of this device has been reported in several conditions and with a change in cannulae configuration it can be used in acute myocardial infarction, post-LVAD implantation, pulmonary hypertension, severe acute mitral regurgitation, and cardiac rejections after heart transplantation [34, 62]. This device has also been successfully used for post-myocardial infarction interventricular septum defect, allowing time for left ventricular recovery and definitive surgical repair [63].

The Berlin Heart INCOR (Berlin Heart GmbH., Berlin, Germany) is an implantable VAD that has an active magnetically levitated rotor. It is implanted below the diaphragm in an abdominal pump pocket and due to the size, it is not viewed as being suitable for less invasive implantation methods. Despite its designs, the initial results were undermined due to issues with the design of the inflow cannula causing high rates of embolic complications. The first in human use was in 2002. However, recent results with new designs have shown improved results with respect to GI bleeding and *de novo* pump thrombosis [64].

The Ventracor (is no longer trading) was developed in 1997 with the first in human use in 2003. Approximately 450 devices were implanted before the company ceased trading in 2009 [55].

The Arrow CorAide left ventricular assist system (LVAS) (Arrow International, Reading, PA, USA) is a continuous flow left ventricular assist device, as a bridge to transplantation or recovery as well as destination therapy in patients with New York Heart Association (NYHA) class IV heart failure. Its use has been limited to clinical trials and was originally developed at the Cleveland Clinic. The first patient was implanted in May 2003. It was the first third-generation magnetically levitated pump to be included in a clinical trial [65].

3. Temporary and durable mechanical circulatory support

With the progress in comprehensive evaluation, and diagnostic and therapeutic approaches in patients with heart failure, device selection has become the cornerstone for improving outcomes. Guidelines in the acute and chronic management of cardiovascular failure have incorporated importance to categorize individuals based on the severity and acuity of the disease. Therefore, the Interagency Registry for Mechanically Assisted Circulatory Support (INTERMACS) was founded in 2005 to summarize the clinical outcome profiles of patients with advanced stage HF who receive a MCS device. This classification encompasses seven progressive clinical profiles within the NYHA class III and IV functional status. Short-term or temporary devices are generally recommended to provide uni- or bi-ventricular assistance to patients with cardiogenic shock, decompensated heart failure, cardiac arrest, or high-risk percutaneous coronary interventions. Therefore, these devices are typically employed for bridging patients to transplantation, recovery, or bridge-to-decision. Models of temporary support have included the intra-aortic balloon pump, the Impella devices (AbioMed, Danvers, MA, USA), the TandemHeart (LivaNova, London, England, UK), the Rotaflow (Maquet), the CentriMag/PediMag (Abbott), and the veno-arterial extracorporeal membrane oxygenation. Durable devices have been divided as previously described, first-, second-, and third-generation devices based on the flow mechanics. Many of these devices have evolved to provide better features such a smaller size, improved biological compatibility, and an overall reduction in costs and adversity.

4. Current trends in mechanical circulatory support

It has been estimated that survival rates in patients with continuous flow devices are 81% and 70% at 1- and 2-year post-implantation, respectively. Additionally, survival trends showed that outcomes are more satisfactory in VADs used for BTT than those in the DT cohorts. Nevertheless, even in the DT population, which inherently possesses greater comorbidities that contraindicate them for HT, long-term outcomes are still excellent exhibiting 68% overall survival at 2 years [66]. The Heartmate III recently achieved ~80% in the primary composite outcome of survival without disabling stroke or reoperation at 2 years [67]. Beyond implantation and the perioperative risks, this difference primarily resulted from a substantial reduction in the incidence of pump-related thromboembolic phenomena and reoperation due to device malfunctioning. Furthermore, data suggest that proactive implantation of VADs in patients with heart failure (INTERMACS classes 4–7) has excellent outcomes with a survival rate in the 80–95% range 1 year after implantation. Certainly, technological advances have made a significant difference in the last decades. In addition, at many centers, the selection of appropriate candidates for mechanical support has been developed to incorporate multidisciplinary evaluation before implantation. The harmonization of this approach provides meaningful benefits, as some studies have identified numerous comorbidities that are associated with poor outcomes. Such factors include limited life expectancy, active malignancy, multisystemic end-stage organ dysfunction, severe infections, hematologic dyscrasias, and anatomical and psychological components [66].

5. Conclusion

Over the last decades, there have been revolutionary developments in mechanical support. Although patients with chronic heart failure exhibit improved survivorship with the application of evidence-based medical therapies, VADs are superior to medical therapy for improving survival among patients with advanced heart failure with reduced ejection fraction [18]. This topic is important because estimates reveal that over 18 million persons are diagnosed with heart failure in the United States and Europe at present [17]. Furthermore, heart failure is far more prevalent in older age groups, reaching 4.3% among persons aged 65–70 years in 2012, and is projected to increase steadily, reaching 8.5% in the US by the year 2030 [17].

For individuals with refractory heart failure requiring transplantation, it has been estimated that a VAD is used as a bridge to transplantation in approximately 9% of children and 25% of adult patients The shortage of donor organs and the expanding pool of patients with heart failure have led to growing interest in mechanical circulatory support; fortunately, we have observed meaningful and positive trends from the incorporation of MCS over the past five decades. We commend all those individuals who have been at the forefront of these developments and equally acknowledge those with behind-the-scenes contributions to this field.

As of today, this modality has been successfully expanded to employ MCS as bridge-to-transplant, bridge-to-recuperation, or destination therapy. However, following the withdrawal of HVAD from the global market in June of 2021, we are currently left with a reduced armamentarium for managing patients with advanced heart failure with reduced ejection fraction, particularly in the pediatric population. Therefore, shifting the paradigm to advance device miniaturization, improving surgical implantation techniques, and effectively reducing adverse events would be of greatest value in the following decades to further advance the field of mechanical circulation. An integrative alliance among technology companies, healthcare practitioners, and researchers is paramount to promoting education, innovation, and accessibility.

Acknowledgements

This publication was supported by the St. Jude Pediatric Research Recruitment Support Fund (R079700270) hosted by H.R.M.

Conflict of interest

The authors declare no conflict of interest.

Appendices and nomenclature

ACTION	Advanced Cardiac Therapies Improving Outcomes Network
BiVAD	biventricular assist device
BTR	bridge to recovery
BTT	bridge to transplantation
Circulatory support	
CPB	cardiopulmonary bypass
DT	destination therapy
EUROMACS	European Registry for Patients Assisted with Mechanical
FDA	Food and Drug Administration
HF	heart failure
HVAD	HeartWare Ventricular Assist Device
INTERMACS	Interagency Registry for Mechanically Assisted Circulatory
Support	
LVAD	left ventricular assist device
LVAS	left ventricular assist system
MCS	mechanical circulatory support

MOMENTUM 3	Multicenter Study of MagLev Technology in Patients Undergoing Mechanical Circulatory Support Therapy with HeartMate 3
NHLBI	National Hearts, Lung, and Blood Institute
NIH	National Institutes of Health
RV	right ventricle
RVAD	right ventricular assist device
STS	Society of Thoracic Surgeons
TAH	total artificial heart
US SUSTAIN Trial	A Study Evaluating Safety and Effectiveness of the DuraHeart Left Ventricular Assist System in Bridge to Transplant Patients
VAD	ventricular assist device

Author details

Hugo Martinez[1*], Neely R. Alberson[2], Jarot J. Guerra[3] and Ismael A. Salas De Armas[3]

1 Division of Pediatric Cardiology and Genetics, Le Bonheur Children's Hospital, Heart Institute, The University of Tennessee Health Science Center, Memphis, TN, USA

2 Department of Pediatrics, Le Bonheur Children's Hospital, College of Medicine, Children's Foundation Research Institute, The University of Tennessee Health Science Center, Memphis, TN, USA

3 Department of Advanced Cardiopulmonary Therapies and Transplantation, The University of Texas Health Science Center at Houston, TX, USA

*Address all correspondence to: hmartinez@uthsc.edu

References

[1] Virani SS, Alonso A, Aparicio HJ, Benjamin EJ, Bittencourt MS, Callaway CW, et al. Heart disease and stroke Statistics-2021 update: A report from the American Heart Association. Circulation. 2021;**143**(8):e254-e743

[2] OPTN Organ Procurement and Transplantation Network. 2022. Available from: https://optn.transplant.hrsa.gov/.

[3] Gibbon JH Jr. Application of a mechanical heart and lung apparatus to cardiac surgery. Minnesota Medicine. 1954;**37**(3):171-185; passim

[4] DeBakey ME. Development of mechanical heart devices. The Annals of Thoracic Surgery. 2005;**79**(6):2228

[5] Ensminger SM, Gerosa G, Gummert JF, Falk V. Mechanical circulatory support: Heart failure therapy "in motion". Innovations (Phila). 2016;**11**(5):305-314

[6] Liotta D, Hall CW, Henly WS, Cooley DA, Crawford ES, DeBakey ME. Prolonged assisted circulation during and after cardiac or aortic surgery: Prolonged partial left ventricular bypass by means of intracorporeal circulation. The American Journal of Cardiology. 1963;**12**(3):399-405

[7] Berardi C, Bravo CA, Li S, Khorsandi M, Keenan JE, Auld J, et al. The history of durable left ventricular assist devices and comparison of outcomes: HeartWare, heart mate II, heart mate 3, and the future of mechanical circulatory support. Journal of Clinical Medicine. 2022;**11**(7):2022. DOI: 10.3390/jcm11072022

[8] Barnard CN, The operation. A human cardiac transplant: An interim report of a successful operation performed at Groote Schuur hospital, Cape Town. South African Medical Journal. 1967;**41**(48):1271-1274

[9] Kirklin JK, Naftel DC. Mechanical circulatory support: Registering a therapy in evolution. Circulation. Heart Failure. 2008;**1**(3):200-205

[10] Stewart GC, Givertz MM. Mechanical circulatory support for advanced heart failure: Patients and technology in evolution. Circulation. 2012;**125**(10):1304-1315

[11] Cooley DA, Liotta D, Hallman GL, Bloodwell RD, Leachman RD, Milam JD. Orthotopic cardiac prosthesis for two-staged cardiac replacement. The American Journal of Cardiology. 1969;**24**(5):723-730

[12] Norman JC, Brook MI, Cooley DA, Klima T, Kahan BD, Frazier OH, et al. Total support of the circulation of a patient with post-cardiotomy stone-heart syndrome by a partial artificial heart (ALVAD) for 5 days followed by heart and kidney transplantation. Lancet. 1978;**1**(8074):1125-1127

[13] DeVries WC, Anderson JL, Joyce LD, Anderson FL, Hammond EH, Jarvik RK, et al. Clinical use of the total artificial heart. The New England Journal of Medicine. 1984;**310**(5):273-278

[14] Portner PM, Oyer PE, Pennington DG, Baumgartner WA, Griffith BP, Frist WR, et al. Implantable electrical left ventricular assist systems: Bridge to transplantation and future. The Annals of Thoracic Surgery. 1989;**47**(1):142-150

[15] Han J, Trumble DR. Cardiac assist devices: Early concepts, current

technologies, and future innovations. Bioengineering (Basel). 2019;**6**(1):18. DOI: 10.3390/bioengineering6010018

[16] Rose EA, Gelijns AC, Moskowitz AJ, Heitjan DF, Stevenson LW, Dembitsky W, et al. Long-term use of a left ventricular assist device for end-stage heart failure. The New England Journal of Medicine. 2001;**345**(20):1435-1443

[17] Roger VL. Epidemiology of heart failure: A contemporary perspective. Circulation Research. 2021;**128**(10):1421-1434

[18] Cornwell WK 3rd, Stöhr EJ, BJ MD, Aaronson K, Hayward C, Pal JD. The future of mechanical circulatory support. Circulation. Heart Failure. 2021;**14**(8):e008861

[19] Mancini D, Colombo PC. Left ventricular assist devices: A rapidly evolving alternative to transplant. Journal of the American College of Cardiology. 2015;**65**(23):2542-2555

[20] Goodman D, Stulak J, Rosenbaum AN. Left ventricular assist devices: A historical perspective at the intersection of medicine and engineering. Artificial Organs. 2022;**46**(12):2343-2360

[21] Prinzing A, Herold U, Berkefeld A, Krane M, Lange R, Voss B. Left ventricular assist devices—Current state and perspectives. Journal of Thoracic Disease. 2016;**8**(8):E660-E666

[22] Wu EL, Stevens MC, Pauls JP, Steinseifer U. Chapter 3- first-generation ventricular assist devices. In: Gregory SD, Stevens MC, Fraser JF, editors. Mechanical Circulatory and Respiratory Support. London, UK: Academic Press; 2018. pp. 93-115

[23] Ying GS, Heitjan DF. Prediction of event times in the REMATCH trial. Clinical Trials. 2013;**10**(2):197-206

[24] Wheeldon DR, LaForge DH, Lee J, Jansen PG, Jassawalla JS, Portner PM. Novacor left ventricular assist system long-term performance: Comparison of clinical experience with demonstrated in vitro reliability. ASAIO Journal. 2002;**48**(5):546-551

[25] Dagenais F, Portner PM, Robbins RC, Oyer PE. The Novacor left ventricular assist system: Clinical experience from the Novacor registry. Journal of Cardiac Surgery. 2001;**16**(4):267-271

[26] Mehta SM, Pae WE Jr, Rosenberg G, Snyder AJ, Weiss WJ, Lewis JP, et al. The lion heart LVD-2000: A completely implanted left ventricular assist device for chronic circulatory support. The Annals of Thoracic Surgery. 2001;**71**(Suppl. 3):S156-S154

[27] Nersesian G, Hennig F, Müller M, Mulzer J, Tsyganenko D, Starck C, et al. Temporary mechanical circulatory support for refractory heart failure: The German heart center Berlin experience. Annals of Cardiothoracic Surgery. 2018;**8**(1):76-83

[28] Tominaga Y, Ueno T, Kido T, Kanaya T, Narita J, Ishida H, et al. Bridge to recovery with Berlin heart EXCOR in children <10 kg with dilated cardiomyopathy: A histological analysis. European Journal of Cardio-Thoracic Surgery. 2020;**58**(2):253-260

[29] Adachi I, Burki S, Zafar F, Morales DLS. Pediatric ventricular assist devices. Journal of Thoracic Disease. 2015;**7**(12):2194-2202

[30] Gregory SD, Timms D, Gaddum N, Mason DG, Fraser JF. Biventricular assist devices: A technical review. Annals of Biomedical Engineering. 2011;**39**(9):2313-2328

[31] Samuels LE, Holmes EC, Thomas MP, Entwistle JC 3rd, Morris RJ,

Narula J, et al. Management of acute cardiac failure with mechanical assist: Experience with the ABIOMED BVS 5000. The Annals of Thoracic Surgery. 2001;**71**(Suppl. 3):S67-S65

[32] Morgan JA, Stewart AS, Lee BJ, Oz MC, Naka Y. Role of the Abiomed BVS 5000 device for short-term support and bridge to transplantation. ASAIO Journal. 2004;**50**(4):360-363

[33] Samuels LE, Holmes EC, Hagan K, Gopalan R, Droogan C, Ferdinand F. The Thoratec implantable ventricular assist device (IVAD): Initial clinical experience. The Heart Surgery Forum. 2006;**9**(4):690

[34] Graefe R, Groß-Hardt S. Chapter 4 - second-generation ventricular assist devices. In: Gregory SD, Stevens MC, Fraser JF, editors. Mechanical Circulatory and Respiratory Support. London, UK: Academic Press; 2018. pp. 117-150

[35] Noon GP, Ball JW Jr, Papaconstantinou HT. Clinical experience with BioMedicus centrifugal ventricular support in 172 patients. Artificial Organs. 1995;**19**(7):756-760

[36] Frazier OH, Wampler RK, Duncan JM, Dear WE, Macris MP, Parnis SM, et al. First human use of the Hemopump, a catheter-mounted ventricular assist device. The Annals of Thoracic Surgery. 1990;**49**(2):299-304

[37] Noon GP, Morley D, Irwin S, Benkowski R. Development and clinical application of the micro med DeBakey VAD. Current Opinion in Cardiology. 2000;**15**(3):166-171

[38] Hetzer R, Javier MFDM, Dandel M, Loebe M, Javier Delmo EM. Mechanical circulatory support systems: Evolution, the systems and outlook. Cardiovascular Diagnosis and Therapy. 2021;**11**(1):309-322

[39] Anderson MB, Goldstein J, Milano C, Morris LD, Kormos RL, Bhama J, et al. Benefits of a novel percutaneous ventricular assist device for right heart failure: The prospective RECOVER RIGHT study of the Impella RP device. The Journal of Heart and Lung Transplantation. 2015;**34**(12):1549-1560

[40] Raess DH, Weber DM. Impella 2.5. Journal of Cardiovascular Translational Research. 2009;**2**(2):168-172

[41] Kovacic JC, Kini A, Banerjee S, Dangas G, Massaro J, Mehran R, et al. Patients with 3-vessel coronary artery disease and impaired ventricular function undergoing PCI with Impella 2.5 hemodynamic support have improved 90-day outcomes compared to intra-aortic balloon pump: A sub-study of the PROTECT II trial. Journal of Interventional Cardiology. 2015;**28**(1):32-40

[42] Salas De Armas IA, Patel MK, Patel JA, Akay MH, Marcano J, Kar B, et al. Insertion of Impella 5.5 via the axillary artery graft under fluoroscopic guidance. Operative Techniques in Thoracic and Cardiovascular Surgery. 2021;**26**(3):462-474

[43] Salas de Armas IA, Shirafkan A, Akay MH, Patel J, Patel MK, Marcano J, et al. Transaortic placement of percutaneous mechanical support device via partial sternotomy: Feasible option for unsuitable axillary artery access. Innovations (Phila). 2022;**17**(5):377-381

[44] Zein R, Patel C, Mercado-Alamo A, Schreiber T, Kaki A. A review of the Impella devices. Interventional Cardiology. 2022;**17**:e05

[45] Salas de Armas I, Bergeron A, Bhardwaj A, Patarroyo M, Akay MH, Al Rameni D, et al. Surgically implanted Impella device for patients on

Impella CP support experiencing refractory hemolysis. ASAIO Journal. 2022;**68**(12):e251-e255

[46] Agrawal N, Hameed FR, Kumar S, Akkanti B, Hussain R, Jumean MF, et al. Bridge to decision or destination with Impella 5.0 and 5.5 In cardiogenic shock. Journal of Cardiac Failure. 2022;**28**(Suppl. 5):S74

[47] Selzman CH, Koliopoulou A, Glotzbach JP, McKellar SH. Evolutionary improvements in the Jarvik 2000 left ventricular assist device. ASAIO Journal. 2018;**64**(6):827-830

[48] Gregoric ID, La Francesca S, Myers T, Cohn W, Loyalka P, Kar B, et al. A less invasive approach to axial flow pump insertion. The Journal of Heart and Lung Transplantation. 2008;**27**(4):423-426

[49] Maltais S, Kilic A, Nathan S, Keebler M, Emani S, Ransom J, et al. PREVENtion of heart mate II pump thrombosis through clinical management: The PREVENT multi-center study. The Journal of Heart and Lung Transplantation. 2017;**36**(1):1-12

[50] Imamura T, Narang N, Rodgers D, Nguyen A, Ota T, Song T, et al. Outcomes following left ventricular assist device exchange. Journal of Cardiac Surgery. 2020;**35**(3):591-597

[51] Coyle L, Graney N, Gallagher C, Paliga R, Yost G, Pappas P, et al. Treatment of heart mate II short-to-shield patients with an ungrounded cable: Indications and long-term outcomes. ASAIO Journal. 2020;**66**(4):381-387

[52] Flint KM, Brieke A, Cornwell WK 3rd, Pierce C, Cleveland JC, Pal JD. Heart mate II system controller failure presenting as driveline fault with repeated pump stoppages. Circulation. Heart Failure. 2019;**12**(7):e005738

[53] Fujii Y, Ferro G, Kagawa H, Centola L, Zhu L, Ferrier WT, et al. Is continuous flow superior to pulsatile flow in single ventricle mechanical support? Results from a large animal pilot study. ASAIO Journal. 2015;**61**(4):443-447

[54] Kitamura T, Torii S, Oka N, Horai T, Itatani K, Yoshii T, et al. Seventeen-month-long paracorporeal biventricular mechanical support as a bridge to transplantation for severe dilated cardiomyopathy. Journal of Artificial Organs. 2015;**18**(1):92-94

[55] Foster G. Chapter 5 - third-generation ventricular assist devices. In: Gregory SD, Stevens MC, Fraser JF, editors. Mechanical Circulatory and Respiratory Support. London, UK: Academic Press; 2018. pp. 151-186

[56] Salas De Armas IA, Patel JA, Akay MH, Patel MK, Rajagopal K, Karabulut MN, et al. Off-pump continuous-flow left ventricular assist device implantation. Texas Heart Institute Journal. 2021;**48**(1):e197033. DOI: 10.14503/THIJ-7033

[57] Berardi C, Bravo CA, Li S, Khorsandi M, Keenan JE, Auld J, et al. The history of durable left ventricular assist devices and comparison of outcomes: HeartWare, HeartMate II, HeartMate 3, and the future of mechanical circulatory support. Journal of Clinical Medicine. 2022;**11**(7):2022

[58] Mehra MR, Goldstein DJ, Cleveland JC, Cowger JA, Hall S, Salerno CT, et al. Five-year outcomes in patients with fully magnetically levitated vs axial-flow left ventricular assist devices in

the MOMENTUM 3 randomized trial. JAMA. 2022;**328**(12):1233-1242

[59] Daneshmand MA, Bishawi M, Milano CA, Schroder JN. The HeartMate 6. ASAIO Journal. 2020;**66**(3):e46-e49

[60] Timms D. A review of clinical ventricular assist devices. Medical Engineering & Physics. 2011;**33**(9):1041-1047

[61] Moazami N, Steffen RJ, Naka Y, Jorde U, Bailey S, Murali S, et al. Lessons learned from the first fully magnetically levitated centrifugal LVAD trial in the United States: The dura heart trial. The Annals of Thoracic Surgery. 2014;**98**(2):541-547

[62] Schmack B, Weymann A, Popov AF, Patil NP, Sabashnikov A, Kremer J, et al. Concurrent left ventricular assist device (LVAD) implantation and percutaneous temporary RVAD support via CardiacAssist Protek-duo tandem heart to preempt right heart failure. Medical Science Monitor Basic Research. 2016;**22**:53-57

[63] Gregoric ID, Bieniarz MC, Arora H, Frazier OH, Kar B, Loyalka P. Percutaneous ventricular assist device support in a patient with a postinfarction ventricular septal defect. Texas Heart Institute Journal. 2008;**35**(1):46-49

[64] Iacovoni A, Centofanti P, Attisani M, Verde A, Terzi A, Senni M, et al. Low incidence of gastrointestinal bleeding and pump thrombosis in patients receiving the INCOR LVAD system in the long-term follow-up. The International Journal of Artificial Organs. 2015;**38**(10): 542-547

[65] Saeed D, Arusoglu L, Gazzoli F, Hetzer R, Morshius M, Alloni A, et al. Results of the European clinical trial of arrow CorAide left ventricular assist system. Artificial Organs. 2013;**37**(2):121-127

[66] Han JJ, Acker MA, Atluri P. Left ventricular assist devices. Circulation. 2018;**138**(24):2841-2851

[67] Mehra MR, Cleveland JC Jr, Uriel N, Cowger JA, Hall S, Horstmanshof D, et al. Primary results of long-term outcomes in the MOMENTUM 3 pivotal trial and continued access protocol study phase: A study of 2200 HeartMate 3 left ventricular assist device implants. European Journal of Heart Failure. 2021;**23**(8):1392-1400

Section 2

Cardiac Remodeling Related to Mechanical Circulatory Support

Chapter 2

Myocardial Remodeling with Ventricular Assist Devices

Buyan-Ochir Orgil, Neely R. Alberson, Jeffrey A. Towbin and Enkhsaikhan Purevjav

Abstract

Most prominent functional abnormalities seen in the failing human heart are impaired contraction and slowed rates of relaxation of cardiac cells in the face of increased neurohormonal activation, sustained inflammation, mechanical and volume overload, and progressive maladaptive remodeling of the myocardium. Mechanical circulatory support devices (MCS) improve cardiac function and outcomes of patients with end-stage heart failure, allowing to bridge to heart transplantation and permitting the removal of MCS device as a bridge to recovery, in some patients with the sufficient recovery of heart function. Numerous reports have demonstrated favorable myocardial recovery and reverse remodeling after prolonged ventricular unloading by MCS. Ventricular unloading by MCS leads to a decreased concentration of peripheral natriuretic peptides in plasma, reduction in cardiac cytokines, kinases, collagens, and proteins involved in hypertrophy, fibrosis, programmed cell death, and necrosis in the heart. This chapter will summarize and review the effects and underlying mechanisms of myocardial remodeling during prolonged MCS in patients with end-stage heart failure. The mechanisms of myocardial recovery are multifactorial and remain to be further explored on cellular, organ, and systems levels.

Keywords: ventricular assist device, mechanical unloading, reverse remodeling, myocardial recovery, mechanical circulatory support devices (MCS)

1. Introduction

Cardiovascular diseases (CVDs) were responsible for an estimated 17.8 million deaths globally in 2017 and half of all people diagnosed with heart failure (HF) die within 5 years of diagnosis [1]. The major cause for CVD morbidity and mortality is HF, a complex clinical syndrome caused by many CV and other diseases that impairs the ability of the ventricle to fill with or eject blood. The key pathophysiological features involved in the development of HF are hypertrophy, fibrosis, apoptosis/necrosis, microvasculature and extracellular matrix (ECM) abnormalities, and disturbances in electrophysiologic, adrenergic, and angiotensin signaling. Currently, heart transplantation is the gold standard treatment of patients with end-stage HF and the current 10-year survival rates of heart transplant recipients reach 53% [2].

During the last decades, mechanical circulatory support (MCS) devices with ventricular assist devices (VAD) have improved the outcomes of patients with advanced and end-stage HF, becoming a cornerstone therapy to bridge those patients to heart transplantation or recovery [3–7]. The synopsis of structural and molecular changes in the heart underlying the improved cardiac function after VAD implantation is called "reverse cardiac remodeling." Extensive investigations have been utilized to understand how the heart remodels to mechanical and volume unloading during MCS in a facet of stabilized neurohormonal and inflammatory responses [8–10]. MCS therapies lead to the improvement of HF symptoms with normalized cardiac size and shape with simultaneous biological remodeling on gene, molecular, cellular, and tissue levels [11–13]. Myocardial recovery is associated with improvements in structural, sarcomeric, sarcolemmal, and calcium handling-associated proteins expression and function [14–16]. Mechanical unloading has been shown to increase collagen cross-linking and myocardial stiffness [17], alter mitochondrial and metabolic processes [18], and promote repair and regeneration [19]. Moreover, studies focused on understanding the roles of biomarkers of neurohormonal activation, oxidative stress, and systemic inflammation pathways in patients with VAD support have identified a subset of vulnerable patients with risks of developing adverse events fostering the development of innovative applications of combined MSC and pharmacological agents [20, 21]. As a destination therapy MSC is critical in patients with the favorable restoration of cardiac function and this regenerative therapeutic strategy becomes a desirable alternative to heart transplantation [22]. Herein, we review and summarize research studies focused on understanding the roles of neurohormonal signaling, inflammation, signal transduction, cellular and subcellular remodeling, and transcriptional regulation in the failing human heart before and after MCS therapy.

2. Neurohormonal remodeling during LVAD therapy

HF is a highly complex clinical syndrome characterized by cardinal symptoms due to structural and/or functional abnormality of the heart, resulting in elevated intracardiac pressures and/or inadequate cardiac output [23]. The clinical symptoms of HF develop and progress through prolonged dyshomeostasis in the heart in response to various stressors, which include alterations of regulatory neurohormonal systems associated with the release of natriuretic peptides, proinflammatory cytokines as well as activations of the sympathetic nervous system (SNS), which in turn activates the renin-angiotensin-aldosterone system (RAAS) [8]. Some of these alterations appear to be reversible by VAD treatment in response to a decrease in cardiac pressure, volume overload, and ventricular wall tension and stretch [24]. These events lead to reduced cardiomyocyte hypertrophy, improved coronary perfusion, and decreased chronic ischemia in the heart [25]. Therefore, mechanical unloading of the failing heart by LVADs, coupled with neurohormonal and anti-inflammatory therapy, may further promote reverse remodeling and recovery of myocardial function.

2.1 Natriuretic peptides

The natriuretic peptide family consists of atrial natriuretic peptide (ANP), brain natriuretic peptide (BNP), and C-type natriuretic peptide (CNP) [26]. Under normal conditions, ANP is produced in the atrium and BNP is synthesized primarily by the ventricles in response to cardiac mechanical stretch. Circulating in the plasma, ANP and BNP play compensatory diuretic roles by decreasing salt and water retention and inhibiting vasoconstrictor peptides. In contrast to ANP, levels of BNP are significantly elevated in plasma of HF patients in response to chronic volume overload and BNP concentration correlates with the status of ventricular dysfunction with high concentrations predicting poor long-term survival. Support with VAD in patients with end-stage HF reduces the myocardial wall stress and thereby may change BNP levels in the heart. Sodian *et al.* studied 21 patients with nonischemic cardiomyopathy on VAD support and demonstrated a significant decrease in BNP levels in plasma after initiation of MCS, reaching normal levels within the first week after VAD implantation [27]. Especially, an early decrease of BNP in plasma was indicative of cardiac function recovery during VAD support. The significant decrease in BNP serum concentration after VAD support coincides with a decrease in *BNP* messenger RNA (mRNA) and protein expression in the heart of patients with severe HF supported by VAD. They also showed a decrease in BNP production not only by cardiomyocytes, but also by endothelial cells, T cells, and macrophages infiltrating the heart [28].

ANP and BNP also exert local antihypertrophic, antifibrotic, and lusitropic effects in the heart *via* their interactions with guanylyl cyclase-A receptor (CG-AR) [29]. Comparative analysis of cardiac *ANP* and *BNP* mRNAs expression in patients with HF revealed normalization of *ANP*, *BNP*, and the NP-metabolizing *NPR-C* receptor after VAD support, while *GC-AR* mRNA expression levels remained intact, suggesting that reverse remodeling is associated with the local protective effects of ANP and BNP.

In chronic HF, expression of ANP and BNP serves as clinical markers of cardiac hypertrophy, decompensation, hypertension, and myocardial infarction. Acute coronary syndromes are linked with the expression of chromogranin A (CgA), CD56/NCAM (neural cell adhesion molecule), and endothelin-1 (ET-1) [30, 31]. Investigation of 33 paired myocardial and plasma samples demonstrated significantly increased ANP, BNP, and CgA in congestive HF (CHF) patients before LVAD support, and all of these indicators were significantly decreased by VAD support [32]. Concentrations of plasma ANP and BNP also depend on different types of devices and durations of MCS. The time courses of ANP and BNP concentration have been studied in patients supported by Thoratec (8 patients), TCI Heartmate (6 patients), Novacor (7 patients), and Lionheart (3 patients) by Milting *et. al* [33]. All patients supported with Novacor, and some patients supported by TCI Heartmate, showed a steady decrease in plasma BNP levels, reaching normal ranges at 30 to 50 days. In contrast, only few patients supported by Thoratec or Lionheart reached normal BNP plasma values during the entire duration of support, suggesting recognition of different time points in ANP and BNP decrease among various types of devices when weaning from MCS in patients without heart transplant is suggested.

In pediatric cohort, it has been demonstrated that BNP and N-terminal pro-BNP (NT-proBNP) were modified differently by MCS compared to adults, showing an increase up to 1 day after VAD implant with a subsequent decrease to the pre-VAD levels in one month. Another pediatric study found levels of BNP and NT-pro-BNP correlated with severity and unfavorable outcomes of acute decompensated HF and an incremental increase of those peptides within 48 hours of admission predicted the need for MCS [34]. Short-term VAD support in children with severe HF significantly decreased BNP levels in plasma from pre-VAD to post-VAD and reduced markers of apoptosis [35].

2.2 Renin angiotensin aldosterone system

Reduced blood supply causes renal hypoperfusion and stimulation of SNS and RAAS [36]. The key molecule that mediates RAAS activation is angiotensin II (Ang II), a potent vasoconstrictor. In early stages of HF, RAAS activation functions as a compensatory mechanism to increase cardiac output. However, with the HF progression, RAAS activation plays a detrimental role in myocardial ischemia, hypertrophy, and arrhythmia [37]. In end-stage HF, G-protein-coupled receptors (GPCRs) of RAAS, such as Ang receptors, AT1R and AT2R, are downregulated, while angiotensin-converting enzymes (ACE and ACE2), GPCR kinase (GRK), and β-arrestin are upregulated [38]. Following VAD support, a significant downregulation of Ang I, ACE2, GRK, and β-arrestin has been documented, while AT2R, JNK, and p38 were upregulated, indicating divergent and incomplete molecular reverse remodeling. Combined MCS with neurohormonal blockade drug therapy (NHBDT) improved survival and reduced adverse cardiac events in HF [39]. For example, ACE inhibition (ACEI) during VAD support was linked with decreased Ang II, cardiac collagen content, and myocardial stiffness [17, 40], demonstrating the pathophysiological benefits of combined therapy compared with VAD support alone. The ISHLT Mechanically Assisted Circulatory Support (IMACS) registry suggested positive effects for ACEI and angiotensin II receptor blockers (ARBs) therapy in adult HF patients with VAD implantation [41]. Among patients treated with an ACEI/ARB, significantly lower risk of cardiovascular death, gastrointestinal bleeding, and levels of creatinine has been demonstrated compared to those in patients treated with mineralocorticoid receptor antagonist (MRA).

3. Inflammation and cytokines

3.1 Tumor necrosis factor-alpha

Reports on inflammatory profiles in HF patients and LVAD recipients have recently been comprehensively summarized by Radley *et al.* [42]. Tumor necrosis factor-alpha (TNF-α) is a protein expressed in the myocardium that stimulates cardiac growth and cell death [43, 44]. High levels of TNF-α are found in patients with severe HF [45]. Expression of *TNF-α* mRNA and protein were both elevated in the heart and serum of VAD candidates with severe HF [46]. Moreover, interleukin 1 beta (IL-1β), IL-6, procaspase-9, and active caspase-9 were increased in the heart of those deteriorating patients who required VAD support. Torre-Amione *et al.* reported that prolonged MCS results in significant reductions in intracardiac TNF-α, with a greater reduction in myocardial TNF-α in VAD-treated patients with recovered cardiac function *versus* those who required cardiac transplantation [43].

3.2 Metallothionein

Metallothionein (MT) is a highly conserved cytokine-inducible protein whose role is the detoxification of heavy metals through the regulation of their metabolism [47]. High metal affinity to cadmium (Cd) of MT in renal tissue plays a major role in the kinetics and balance between CdMT and non-bound Cd, which is highly neurotoxic [48]. A study of heart transplant patients by Baba *et al.* demonstrated that MT expression correlated with IL-6 elevation in blood vessels and a decrease in plasma IL-2 [49].

Moreover, MT expression was associated with lower fractional shortening, increase in LV end-systolic diameter, and lower mean arterial pressure in the absence of rejection in transplant patients, implicating the role of MT in cellular stress response. Further immunohistochemical studies by the same group demonstrated a decrease of MT-positive cardiomyocytes and vessels in the subendocardial and subepicardial regions of the myocardium in 17 HF patients during prolonged VAD compared to pre-VAD state [50]. In addition, ventricular unloading leads to regression of cellular hypertrophy and a reversal of MT expression in the failing heart, suggesting the remodeling process with reduction of MT expression is due to diminished wall stress and improved blood supply. The authors also observed that MT reactivity was substantially lower in the hearts of patients supported longer than 88 days as compared to patients supported less than 88 days [50].

3.3 C-reactive protein and interleukins

C-reactive protein (CRP) is a protein that is produced in response to the release of pro-inflammatory cytokines when the body is in an inflammatory condition [51]. Patients with end-stage HF have almost 8-fold higher levels of circulating CRP (cCRP) in serum compared to normal references [52]. Batra *et al.* studied pre- and post-implant VAD patients and found that one-third of post-VAD patients have persistently high CRP levels. They concluded that high CRP levels are linked with high mortality risk and a higher possibility of having a stroke during VAD support. Longer VAD therapy (60 days after implantation) resulted in a 50% reduction of CRP levels compared to pre-VAD values, suggesting improved inflammatory status over time [53].

Interleukins (IL) are a group of small molecules and peptides secreted by a wide variety of body cells or cytokines that function in cellular signaling and communication. Serum levels of members of IL-1 family cytokines, IL-1β and IL-33, are highly elevated in HF and remained elevated after MCS [54]. Increased expression of IL-1β and correlated patterns of IL-1 receptors indicate enhanced IL-1β signaling in MCS patients, while expression of IL-33 correlates with CRP plasma levels in HF, but not in patients on MCS. Suppression of tumorigenicity 2 (ST2) is a receptor of IL-33 and coupling of IL-33 with its ST2 receptor (IL-33/ST2) triggers danger-associated cellular responses playing a pivotal role in tissue repair in many organs [55]. In the heart, IL-33 is expressed by activated cardiac fibroblasts and cardiomyocytes during cardiac stretch and then is released into the extracellular matrix (ECM), promoting cell survival by blocking pro-fibrotic intracellular signaling [56, 57]. A significant decrease in soluble ST2 (sST2) levels was observed in end-stage HF patients after VAD implantation, suggesting a lessening of fibrosis and inflammation [58]. Levels of other cytokines, including IL-6 and IL-8, were also linked to the severity of clinical course in end-stage HF patients and correlated with outcome after VAD implantation [59]. A significant correlation of those cytokines was also found with ET-1 and relaxin (RLX)-2, the vasoactive mediators involved in neurohormonal system responses in VAD-supported HF patients [60]. Elevated levels of galectin-3 (GAL-3) were associated with the severity of HF and dynamic changes in GAL-3 levels predicted post-VAD survival [61]. Although unloading with continuous-flow LVAD results in a decrease of GAL-3 levels early post-implant, GAL-3 levels become elevated after 6 months of VAD implantation [61, 62], suggesting that levels of GAL-3 may represent a higher risk of death in HF patients with long-term VAD support.

4. Myocardial remodeling during VAD support

The myocardium consists of cardiomyocytes, composing nearly 56% of the adult heart, fibroblasts (27%), endothelial cells (7%), smooth muscle cells (10%), and various immune cells that transiently reside in the ECM [63]. These cell types are important in preserving normal cardiac function and morphology. The cells interact with each other using reciprocally secreted auto and paracrine factors, secretion of which is regulated by numerous molecules-messengers involving integrins, ET-1, BMPs, PECAM-1, VE-cadherin, VEGF, and TGFβ [64, 65]. Engineered heart tissue (EHT), created *in vitro* by seeding decellularized porcine myocardial sections with primary cardiomyocytes and fibroblasts isolated from neonatal rat ventricular myocardium or with cardiomyocytes derived from human induced pluripotent stem cells (hiPSC), is a novel platform to study cardiac remodeling [66]. Characterization of EHTs demonstrated gradual normalization of stress-free tissue length after mechanical unloading and suggested that actomyosin contraction in cardiomyocytes and activity of fibroblasts may play crucial roles in reverse remodeling after mechanical unloading.

4.1 Cardiac fibroblasts and fibrosis

Cardiac fibrosis in the failing heart is a final product of a series of biomechanical, molecular, and cellular changes that causes an imbalanced increase in ECM production and decreased ECM degradation [67]. The resultant increase in ECM deposition is accompanied by inflammatory and fibrotic scar formation in the interstitial and perivascular areas of the myocardium, interfering with the normal array of cardiomyocytes along with the disturbing supply of oxygen and nutrients to the myocardium. Moreover, cardiac fibrosis triggers further pathological remodeling and functional decline of the heart [68]. According to Tseng *et al.*, an increase in inflammation and fibrosis in the failing heart was associated with an increase in sST2 levels [58]. Synthesis and degradation of collagens I and III are highly regulated processes in human cardiac ECM. Collagen I is a major collagen component establishing the myocyte-collagen matrix, while collagen III contributes to elasticity, and changes in content may influence LV stiffness and size [69]. In HF, predominantly increased accumulation of collagens I and III in ECM results in cardiomyocyte injury, cardiac fibrosis, and the release of collagen-derived peptides into circulation [70]. Bruckner *et al.* recorded a significant decrease in intracardiac TNF-α, collagen I (by 66%), and collagen III (62%) in post-VAD myocardial samples of 18 patients compared to their pre-VAD levels [71]. They also found a decrease in cardiomyocyte size by 26% at post-VAD, demonstrating favorable reverse remodeling in cardiac hypertrophy.

Insulin-like growth factor I (IGF-1), released preferentially from cardiac fibroblasts, functions to negatively regulate atrophy and apoptosis, and stimulate cardiac repair by interacting with stromal cell-derived factor (SDF) [19]. SDF induces IGF-1 expression in cardiac myocytes *in vitro*. Patients with VAD support combined with β2-AR agonist clenbuterol have shown elevated *IGF-1* mRNA at the time of VAD explantation relative to the time of LVAD implantation [72].

4.2 Extracellular matrix remodeling

Matrix metalloproteinases (MMPs) degrade the ECM, while tissue inhibitors of MMPs (TIMPs) prevent the ECM degradation during repair process of damaged tissues and cells. There are four variants of TIMPs that selectively inhibit different types of MMPs [73]. Typically, TIMP1 and MMP1 are increased in patients with deteriorating HF [74]. The increased ratio of MMP-1 to TIMP-1 in DCM has been shown to be almost normalized after LVAD, favoring decreased collagen degradation [17]. Felkin *et al.* found that high myocardial MMP1 and MMP8 expression is associated with high collagen content and increased IL-6 and IL-1β expression in HF patients requiring VAD support [75]. After VAD support, expression of *MMP-2* mRNA and active MMP-2 protein has been shown to be significantly increased compared to pre-VAD ($P < 0.01$), which was associated with a reduction of collagen IV content in the cardiomyocyte basement membrane. Furthermore, this was associated with a decrease in the thickness of cardiomyocyte membrane as revealed by electron microscopy [76]. MCS support increases collagen cross-linking and the ratio of collagen I to III in the heart as a result of decreased tissue MMP-1-to-TIMP-1 ratio and increased myocardial Ang I and II levels that stimulate ECM synthesis [17]. Therapy with ACEI drugs decreased Ang II levels and myocardial collagen content, resulting in enhanced myocardial recovery during VAD support [40]. In elderly patients with end-stage HF, VAD therapy is associated with decreased collagen turnover and cross-linking and increased tissue Ang II, whereas combined VAD and ACEI therapy normalizes LV end-diastolic pressure-volume relationships [77].

4.3 Endothelial and vasculature remodeling

A gene ontology (GO) analysis implicated endothelial to mesenchymal transition (EndoMT) and *vice versa* (MEndoT) pathways in human end-stage HF based on dual expressed VE-Cadherin endothelial and FSP-1 mesenchymal markers [78]. Gene expression analysis of 19 paired pre-VAD and post-VAD human heart samples by Hall *et al.* revealed differential expression of neuropilin-1, *FGF9*, *Sprouty1*, SDF1, and endomucin, the genes involved in the regulation of vascular networks [79]. In addition, a significant downregulation of GATA-4 binding protein, a critical mediator of myocyte hypertrophy, was observed in these heart samples following mechanical unloading. Drakos *et al.* observed an increased density of endothelial cells by 33% and decreased microvascular lumen area (36%) in post-VAD *vs* pre-VAD myocardial samples of patients with chronic HF ($n = 15$). This was associated with the activation of endothelial cells evidenced by ultrastructural and immunohistochemical analysis [80]. In agreement with these findings, a significant increase in interstitial and total collagen content without structural changes in cardiomyocytes was suggestive of increased fibrosis accompanied by regression of cardiomyocyte hypertrophy.

4.4 Reversal of cardiac hypertrophy

The myocardium is typically subjected to three types of mechanical loading during every heartbeat, including cyclic stretch, static stretch, and shear stress, generated by blood flow and an increase in chamber volume and pressure. Cardiomyocytes are sensitive to mechanical stress, which is transduced to molecular transduction signaling by biomechanical sensors. Comparative analysis of cardiomyocyte size in pre- and post-VAD patients demonstrated a decrease of 26% (33.1 ± 1.32 to 24.4 ± 1.64 μm, $P < 0.001$) in all patients studied [71]. Long-term VAD support resulted in a 28% reduction in myocyte volume, 20% reduction in cell length, 20% reduction in cell width, and 32% reduction in cell length-to-thickness ratio [81]. Another study examined the effects of continuous-flow VAD on cardiomyocyte size and demonstrated that cardiomyocyte cross-sectional area decreased after VAD, but not beyond that of normal donor hearts [82]. Electron microscopy, cardiac glycogen content, and echocardiographic assessment also did not suggest myocardial atrophy in post-VAD patients. Consistent with these findings, no upregulation of pro-atrophic genes and proteins of the ubiquitin-proteasome system (UPS) and no t-tubule pathologies have been demonstrated.

Myostatin (also called gdf-8) is a potent inhibitor of skeletal muscle growth from the TGF-β family and is secreted by cardiac muscle and adipocytes in response to pathological stress, such as myocardial infarction or obesity [83]. Myostatin has been shown to mediate the regression of cellular hypertrophy after unloading with LVAD support [84]. The nuclear factor (NF)-κB superfamily of transcription factors carries out broad functions by regulating immune cell maturation, cell survival, and inflammation in many cell types [85]. In the heart, NF-κB is shown to be cardioprotective during acute injury, however, prolonged activation of NF-κB enhances the release of TNF-α, IL-1, and IL-6 cytokines, triggering chronic inflammation, hypertrophy, and cell death [86, 87]. After VAD support, the NF-κB DNA-binding activity decreases in failing human hearts and this process has been associated with a decrease in cardiomyocyte diameter [88].

Several kinases such as mitogen-activated protein kinase (MAPK or MEK), ERK (extracellularly regulated kinase), AKT (protein kinase B, PKB), GSK-3b (glycogen synthase kinase-3 beta), JNK (c-Jun NH2-terminal kinase) and p38 are involved in the development of cardiac hypertrophy *via* kinase-mediated signal transduction pathways [89]. After VAD support, significantly decreased activities of ERKs and AKT were seen in failing hearts, while the activity of GSK-3β was increased [90]. These changes were associated with a decrease in TUNEL-positivity and myocyte diameter. The disparity in the regulation of MAPK activity with a concomitant decrease in ERK and JNK1/2 activities and an increase in p38 activity after VAD support has been also reported [91].

Osteopontin (OPN) is a pleiotropic extracellular signal-regulated bone sialoprotein. Expression and activity of OPN are increased in myocardial tissues in accordance with the severity of HF [92]. Levels of *OPN* mRNA in heart biopsy specimens decreased significantly after VAD support, while OPN protein remained intact [93]. Moreover, VAD support induced a decrease of OPN levels in the plasma of some patients with VAD support, whereas OPN plasma levels were reduced significantly in all patients after a heart transplant.

4.5 Cardiomyocyte apoptosis

While MCS improves the survival of end-stage HF patients by reversing many biological processes activated during progression of HF, the reports on modulation of apoptotic cell death in response to VAD remain controversial. Prescimone *et al.* found a significant increase of Bax (pro-apoptotic), Bcl-2 (pro-apoptotic), and Hsp72 (antiapoptotic) molecules and a mild increase in cardiac caspase (Casp)-3 activity in post-VAD hearts compared to pre-VAD, suggesting involvement of mitochondria in apoptotic signaling [94]. The authors also found an increase in Casp-1 after VAD implant in HF patients and lack of apoptotic nuclei [95]. Conversely, Francis *et al.* found Bcl-2 being downregulated after VAD implant [96]. Another study found no significant differences in Bcl-2, while autophagy markers such as beclin-1, autophagy-related gene 5 (Atg5), and microtubule-associated protein-1 light chain-3 (LC3) were all significantly decreased in response to unloading [97]. Moreover, Bedi *et al.*

observed a highly variable expression of Fas among patients who had undergone MSC therapy [98]. Fas, also called Apo-1 or CD95, is a membrane receptor recognizing Fas ligand (Fas-L) and Fas/Fas-L coupling initiates an apoptotic cell death through the activation of caspase cascade in the heart [99]. Although apoptotic DNA fragmentation was attenuated in the myocardium, expression of antiapoptotic *Bcl-XL* and *FasExo6Del/Fas* genes was dependent on the duration of MCS [100]. Overall, no significant differences in number of TUNEL-positive cells between pre- and post-VAD samples have been reported by several groups [96, 97, 101, 102].

Abnormal Ca^{2+} cycling in HF triggers activation of UPS with an increase of binding immunoglobulin protein (BiP), eukaryotic initiation factor (eIF2α), and X-box binding protein 1 (XBP1) [103]. MCS support significantly decreases the levels of BiP and XBP1 and phosphorylation of eIF2α [104]. Moreover, a decrease in apoptosis observed during short-term VAD support has been associated with a decrease in phosphorylation of SMAD2 (mothers against decapentaplegic homolog 2), however, a long-term VAD support increased apoptosis and fibrosis in the heart *via* enhanced SMAD2 signaling and increased phosphorylation of HDAC4 (histone deacetylase 4) [101].

4.6 Cardiomyocyte regeneration

Diploid cardiomyocytes that are abundant in animal heart have a substantial capacity for cardiac repair and regeneration [105]. In human failing heart, polyploidy of cardiomyocytes is often observed as a precondition of heart hypertrophy [106], suggesting that cardiomyocyte polyploidization in HF may be associated with regeneration [107]. A study by Wohlschlaeger *et al.* demonstrated a marked reduction in the size of cardiomyocyte nuclei and in ratios between number of nuclei and cardiac myocytes after implantation of VAD [108]. They also reported a significant decrease in DNA content and reduction of polyploid cardiomyocytes in 23 myocardial samples studied after VAD, suggesting a decline in protein synthesis. On the contrary, an increase in the number of diploid cardiomyocytes was seen by other groups in post-VAD samples [108]. The decrease in polyploidy and increase in diploidy in response to MCS suggested an abundance of diploid cardiomyocytes going through cell cycle progression with the completion of mitosis or increase in stem cells. Prolonged MCS unloading increased the number of cardiomyocytes positive for phosphorylated histone H3 and Aurora B and this was associated with a decrease in cardiomyocyte size and mitochondrial content [109].

4.7 Transcriptional changes during VAD therapy

Accumulating evidence shows that the changes in transcriptome and metabolome profiles associated with HF persist in the reverse-remodeled myocardium despite apparent normalization on organ and cellular levels [110]. To identify transcriptional adaptations in failing and VAD-supported hearts, a comprehensive transcription analysis was performed in 199 human myocardial samples from nonfailing, failing, and VAD-supported human hearts. Although over 3088 transcripts exhibited alterations in HF samples, the number of differentially expressed genes (DEGs) with greater than or equal to a 2-fold difference was insignificant between HF and post-VAD samples, suggesting that many HF-associated transcriptional changes may have a limited role in regulating cardiac structure and function [111]. Significant elevation in myocardial arginine/glycine amidinotransferase (AGAT) expression is observed in

HF patients and myocardial *AGAT* is one of the DEGs that had a significant decrease during recovery [112]. In HF patients recovering after combination therapy, levels of *AGAT* mRNA decreased by 4.3-fold [$P < 0.001$] and 2.7-fold [$P < 0.005$] in VAD combined and VAD alone groups compared to donors, respectively, and *AGAT* levels returned to normal after recovery. These data highlighted the involvement of elevated local creatine synthesis specific to HF and its reversal during recovery. The genetic response of pediatric myocardium to MCS is distinct with approximately 40% of DEGs compared to adult hearts with VAD support, highlighting the importance of understanding features of reverse remodeling specific to pediatric myocardium to improve clinical strategies and LVAD management in children [113].

In long-term analysis of gene expression, data of patients studied for an average of 3.8 years post-explant revealed a significant association of integrin signaling and its downstream EPAC2 (exchange protein activated by cyclic-AMP2) during recovery of ventricular function by combined LVAD and clenbuterol therapy [20]. Downregulation of EPAC2 that regulates calcium involving cAMP pathway was associated with improvements in cardiac contractility and metabolism [114].

4.8 miRNAs in response to LVAD therapy

MicroRNAs (miRNAs) are small, endogenous noncoding RNAs that regulate posttranscriptional processes by repressing the translation of targeted protein-coding genes *via* binding to the 3' UTRs of mRNAs [115]. Therefore, cardiac miRNAs and circulating miRNAs (c-miRNAs) are promising biomarkers for HF diagnosis and prognosis [116]. Comprehensive microarray profiling of miRNAs and mRNAs, comparing myocardial specimens from adults with end stage HF with VAD and nonfailing hearts, showed upregulation of 28 miRNAs with almost normalization of miRNA profiles by VAD treatment [117]. Cardiac miRNAs have also been compared in 13 HF children at pre-VAD and at the moment of heart transplant (post-VAD) by next-generation sequencing [118]. The investigators found hsa-miR-199b-5p, hsa-miR-19a-3p, and hsa-miR-1246 being differentially expressed at post-VAD compared to that at pre-VAD. The candidate targets of those differentially expressed miRNAs were sarcomeric troponins showing significantly higher post-VAD when compared with pre-VAD values, suggesting that miRNAs can be therapeutically targeted to improve heart function in pediatric HF. Levels of nine c-miRNAs were downregulated and four c-miRNAs were upregulated in the post-VAD samples *vs* pre-VAD levels [119]. In particular, the c-miR-409-3p has been shown to regulate coagulation factor 7 (F7) and F2, suggesting a role of c-miRNA-409-3p in thrombotic events during MCS.

4.9 Beta-adrenergic receptor remodeling

Myocardial beta-adrenergic receptor (β-AR) signaling is severely diminished in failing heart due to increase in phosphorylation of agonist-occupied β-ARs by GRK2 [120, 121]. In chronic HF, VAD support leads to the restoration of cardiac β-AR signaling *via* the reduction of myocardial GRK2 expression and activity [122]. Unloading with VAD normalizes the ability of cardiac muscle to respond to SNS stimulation, reversing the downregulation of β-ARs [123]. Both types of devices, continuous-flow and pulsatile, decreased the expression and activity of GRK2 and normalized neurohormonal homeostasis disturbed with HF [124]. In pediatric HF, VAD treatment also resulted in the recovery of total β-AR and β_1-AR expressions and reversal of several pathologic processes in the heart [125].

4.10 Cyclic guanosine monophosphate

Cyclic guanosine monophosphate (cGMP) is a cyclic nucleotide derived from GTP (guanosine triphosphate) that acts as a second messenger for activation of intracellular protein kinases in response to the binding of membrane-impermeable hormones to the cell membrane [126]. The important components of cGMP signaling include cGMP-dependent protein kinase G (PKG), ANP, BNP, natriuretic peptide receptor A and C (NPR-A and NPR-C, respectively), neprilysin, NOS3, soluble guanylyl cyclase (sGC), and PDE5 [127]. The cGMP-PKG cascade can decrease the level of calcium and alter the expression of glycoprotein IIb/IIIa. Both fluctuations impact the aggregation of platelets within the body [128]. cGMP levels were found to be higher in patients with implanted VAD compared to healthy individuals. According to Grosman-Rimon *et al.*, cGMP was associated with an elevated risk of gastrointestinal (GI) bleeding during LVAD support [128]. The researchers presume that the association between elevated GI bleeding and higher cGMP levels could be due to platelet abnormalities. The study also found significant alterations of the cGMP-PKG pathway (downregulation of ANP, NPR-C, and cGMP) in patients with dilated cardiomyopathy after VAD implant, while the duration of VAD support negatively correlated with expression differences of PKG I, PDE5, and sGC in patients with ischemic cardiomyopathy.

5. Cardiomyocyte intracellular remodeling

5.1 Remodeling of cytoskeletal and sarcomeric proteins

Cytoskeletal proteins are essential for the structure and function of the cardiac myocyte. Stetson *et al.* reported ventricular unloading in humans dynamically changes not only myocardial TNF-α, total collagen, and myocyte size, but also remodels the expression of structural proteins [129]. To understand if myocardial recovery was associated with changes in sarcomeric, nonsarcomeric, and membrane-associated proteins, microarray analysis has been performed on the paired HF samples before and after VAD [16]. Significant increase of lamin A/C, spectrin and integrins (α5 and β5), and decrease of integrins β1, β6, and α7 has been observed at VAD explantation compared to pre-LVAD. Expression of sarcomeric proteins such as β-actin, α-tropomyosin, actinin-α1, and filamin A increased, while troponin T3 and actinin-α2 decreased. Vinculin expression decreased 4.1-fold in the recovered group. Despite decreased cardiomyocyte size post-VAD, severe structural damage in cardiomyocytes persisted with partial improvement in the expression of actin, tropomyosin, troponin C, troponin T, and titin [130]. In pediatric HF, MCS increased the expression of structural proteins, including dystrophin and actin [35]. Furthermore, expression of genes involved in calcium homeostasis, cell differentiation, and growth, including *CNNA1, CDK2B, CSF2, E2F1, EGR1,* and *EGR2*, were normalized after VAD therapy, suggesting an active reverse remodeling process after MCS in pediatric HF.

5.2 Dystrophin remodeling

Dystrophin is a rod-shaped protein encoded by the *DMD* gene located on the X chromosome, the largest gene of 2.4 megabases (Mb) in the human genome [131]. Dystrophin connects the actin and cytoskeleton of muscle fibers to the myocyte membrane at its N-terminus. At the C-terminus, it connects the sarcolemmal complex known as the dystrophin-associated protein complex (DAPC) to the ECM, providing structural support for myocytes. Mutations in *DMD* cause Duchenne and Becker muscular dystrophies [132, 133]. Mutations in genes encoding cytoskeletal and sarcolemmal proteins provide the genetic basis for dilation and contractile dysfunction *via* "final common pathway." Abnormalities in *DMD* such as mutations in the N-terminus of dystrophin or in the cardiac-specific promoter, preferentially affecting cardiac function are associated with X-linked cardiomyopathy [134]. Vatta *et al.* investigated the integrity and response of dystrophin in end-stage dilated or ischemic cardiomyopathy HF patients to VAD therapy and identified disruption of N-terminal dystrophin in 18 HF patients studied [135]. This disruption was shown to be reversible in four patients after VAD support.

5.3 Remodeling in calcium cycling

Regulation of Ca^{2+} cycling is a versatile signaling process that regulates cellular homeostasis in different cell types, including cardiac myocytes [136]. Reduced rates of relaxation and impaired contractile reserve are the major abnormalities seen in the failing heart as a result of disturbances in Ca^{2+} transients [137]. The proteins that regulate cardiomyocyte Ca^{2+} cycling include sarcoplasmic reticulum (SR) Ca^{2+} ATPase (SERCA), ryanodine receptor 2 (RyR2), phospholamban (PLB), and the sarcolemmal Na^{+}/Ca^{2+} exchanger (NCX) [138–140]. Chaudhary *et al.* demonstrated that improvement in cardiac function during LVAD support was associated with a favorable balance between SERCA and NCX, resulting from the isolated decrease in NCX without an increase in SERCA [141]. Reverse remodeling of SERCA2a expression has been shown to be completed by about 20 days of VAD support, while hearts supported by VAD for longer than 40 days have significantly increased relative collagen content [142]. Post-VAD recovery increased SR calcium content and shortened action potential duration due to rapid inactivation in L-type Ca2+ current [15]. Short-term VAD support recovered post-rest potentiation (PRP) response to a level close to that in nonfailing hearts, but recovery of impaired SR Ca^{2+} cycling was dependent on duration MCS [143]. Chronic unloading with recovery of contractile function demonstrated upregulation of *SERCA2a*, *RyR2*, and *NCX* genes after MCS [144]. Recovery of rate-dependent contractility in failing human hearts during early VAD support was associated with faster decay of Ca^{2+} transients, while long-term MCS triggered abnormal Ca^{2+} cycling [101, 143]. Moreover, long-term MCS resulted in significantly increased SMAD2 activity with downstream phosphorylation of Ca^{2+}/calmodulin-dependent protein kinase type-IIδ (CaMKIIδ), myocyte enhancer factor 2 (MEF2), and myostatin. Improvements in the Ca^{2+} handling also depended on the severity of myocardial fibrosis, and ECM pathologies and excessive fibrosis limited the ability to recover [13].

5.4 Mitochondria and metabolism remodeling

Unloading with VAD has been shown to contribute to reverse remodeling of mitochondria and recovery of energy metabolism of the failing heart. In healthy adult hearts, the generation of ATP as a source of energy relies on the oxidation of fatty acids, glucose and lactate in mitochondria, and fatty acid oxidation provides the majority (> 70%) of total ATP [145]. The balance between lactate production and consumption by lactate dehydrogenase (LDH) that converts it to pyruvate, which is then transported by mitochondrial pyruvate carrier (MPC) into the mitochondrial tricarboxylic acid (TCA) cycle is important in producing plentiful ATP. The MPC expression is lower in patients with HF compared to those of non-failing cohorts [146]. Thus, the failing heart runs increased glycolysis and decreased fatty acid oxidation for ATP production and the proportion of glucose oxidation to fatty acid oxidation depends on the severity of HF [147]. The generation of ATP is disturbed in HF with an increased glycolytic pyruvate-derived lactate and a simultaneous decrease in lactate utilization [148]. In addition, the opening of mitochondrial permeability transition pore (mPTP) in HF disrupts the mitochondrial membrane potential and disturbs oxidative phosphorylation pathways for ATP production, causing mitochondrial swelling and inducing apoptotic and necrotic cell death.

MCS improves systemic and cardiac metabolism *via* improvements in fatty acid oxidation, insulin resistance, and reductions in myocardial lipotoxicity through improved activation of the insulin/PI3K/AKT signaling cascade [149]. Significant decrease in long-chain acylcarnitines levels was consistent with improved fatty acid oxidation and utilization during long-term VAD support [150]. Diakos *et al.* reported induction of glycolysis through TCA without a subsequent increase in pyruvate oxidation in post-VAD patients [148], which may be attributed to the poor post-VAD recovery of mitochondrial oxidative capacity. Recently, the same group reported the beneficial cardioprotective effects of induced glycolysis as a result of an increase in rate-limiting enzymes of the pentose-phosphate pathway and 1-carbon metabolism in post-VAD patients [151]. All these have been associated with significantly reduced reactive oxygen species (ROS) and improved mitochondrial density [151, 152]. These metabolic improvements enhanced the glycosylation of α-dystroglycan, which maintains integrity between cytoskeleton and ECM [18]. Moreover, using high-resolution respirometry, a reduction in mitochondrial ROS up to 40% [153] and increased MPC1 abundance and glucose and glucose-6-phosphate levels, particularly, in mechanically unloaded hearts of ischemic HF patients has been demonstrated [154].

Levels of Ca^{2+} in the mitochondrial matrix regulate the activity of kinases and phosphatases involved in ATP production and mitochondrial quality control [155, 156]. In HF, the opening of mPTP not only disrupts the mitochondrial membrane potential but also reduces Ca^{2+} uptake, alters pH, and induces inflammation, leading to necrosis and death of cardiac myocytes [157]. Impaired mitochondrial Ca^{2+} uptake is the result of reduced Ca^{2+} release from SR and stimulates Ca^{2+} –sensitive dehydrogenases of the Krebs cycle [158].

About 20% of the total lipid composition on the mitochondrial inner membrane is constituted by cardiolipin and loss of cardiolipin and tetralinoleoyl-cardiolipin in HF is linked to excessive ROS production and cardiomyocyte apoptosis [159]. During mechanical unloading with LVAD, cardiolipin arrangement normalizes, which in turn, improves mitochondrial coupling [160]. Cellular proteases, such as cathepsins, are involved in the progression of HF. Parallel activation of cathepsins and their inhibitors was observed after VAD support. The expression of cathepsins and their inhibitors was significantly higher in pre-VAD compared to the heart transplant group and VAD induced a further increase in the cathepsin system. Significant positive correlations were observed between cardiac expression of cathepsins and their inhibitors as well as inflammatory cytokines [59, 161].

5.5 Cardiomyocyte signal transduction pathways and signaling

5.5.1 Mitogen-activated protein kinases

There are several cell signal-transduction pathways regulated in the heart in direct response to changes in mechanical loading and stress. The family of MAPKs, such as ERKs, p38, and JNK1/2, are well-characterized signal-transduction pathways [162].

These kinases are involved in the regulation of cell growth, cardiac hypertrophy, and cell death [163, 164]. They are upregulated in patients with HF secondary to ischemic heart disease and cardiomyopathy [165, 166]. The ERKs activity regulates adaptive hypertrophy and prevention of cell death during the early phase of chronic pressure overload in response to stimulation of GPCRs and integrin activation [167]. Mechanical unloading with VAD support resulted in differential regulation of MAPK activity with a significant decrease in the activity of p44/42 ERK and JNK1/2 along with a subsequent increase in p38 activity after LVAD support [91]. The authors explained a decrease in ERK activity is likely due to its decreased phosphorylation at p44/42, while a combination of decreased phosphorylation and expression of JNK1/2 is responsible for decreased JNK1/2 activity in VAD-supported hearts. Activation of AKT regulates cardiac physiological hypertrophy, glucose metabolism, cell death, and angiogenesis [168]. In failing human hearts, a high grade of kinase phosphorylation in all 3 MAPKs and AKT have been observed [166]. After VAD support, ERKs and AKT activities were dramatically decreased in failing hearts, while GSK-3β activities were increased [89].

6. Conclusions

Neurohormonal imbalance, inflammation, apoptosis, and abnormal inter and intracellular signaling and remodeling on molecular and genetic levels are critical processes contributing to adverse events in HF patients. This chapter provides a comprehensive overview of reverse remodeling on neurohormonal, myocardial, and cardiomyocyte intracellular levels in response to MCS in patients with HF. Knowledge about molecular mechanisms of underlying effects of VAD support aid to understand the adverse effects of myocardial unloading and deterioration of patients undergoing VAD therapy. While cardiac reverse remodeling has been correlated with clinical recovery in most post-VAD patients, many of those patients have deteriorated back to the original HF phenotype after LVAD explantation, suggesting the importance of considering a higher degree of myocardial recovery that may persist after device removal [169]. We found a significantly lower number of pediatric reports on clinical and pathological features of reverse remodeling compared to adult HF patients undergoing VAD support. Hence, there is a need for research on pediatric patients with VAD support, so we can better understand features of reverse remodeling specific to pediatric myocardium.

Conflict of interest

None.

Author details

Buyan-Ochir Orgil[1,2], Neely R. Alberson[1,2], Jeffrey A. Towbin[1,2,3]
and Enkhsaikhan Purevjav[1,2*]

1 Heart Institute, University of Tennessee Health Science Center, Memphis, TN, USA

2 Children's Foundation Research Institute, Le Bonheur Children's Hospital, Memphis, TN, USA

3 Pediatric Cardiology, St. Jude Children's Research Hospital, Memphis, TN, USA

*Address all correspondence to: epurevja@uthsc.edu

References

[1] Group, W.C.R.C.W. World Health Organization cardiovascular disease risk charts: Revised models to estimate risk in 21 global regions. The Lancet Global Health. 2019;**7**(10):e1332-e1345

[2] Dolgner SJ et al. Long-term adult congenital heart disease survival after heart transplantation: A restricted mean survival time analysis. The Journal of Heart and Lung Transplantation. 2021;**40**(7):698-706

[3] Miller LW et al. Use of a continuous-flow device in patients awaiting heart transplantation. The New England Journal of Medicine. 2007;**357**(9):885-896

[4] Slaughter MS et al. Advanced heart failure treated with continuous-flow left ventricular assist device. The New England Journal of Medicine. 2009;**361**(23):2241-2251

[5] Rose EA et al. Long-term use of a left ventricular assist device for end-stage heart failure. The New England Journal of Medicine. 2001;**345**(20):1435-1443

[6] Dandel M et al. Long-term results in patients with idiopathic dilated cardiomyopathy after weaning from left ventricular assist devices. Circulation. 2005;**112**(9 Suppl):I37-I45

[7] Frazier OH, Myers TJ. Left ventricular assist system as a bridge to myocardial recovery. The Annals of Thoracic Surgery. 1999;**68**(2):734-741

[8] Liem DA et al. Molecular- and organelle-based predictive paradigm underlying recovery by left ventricular assist device support. Circulation. Heart Failure. 2014;7(2):359-366

[9] Drakos SG et al. Left ventricular assist device unloading effects on myocardial structure and function: Current status of the field and call for action. Current Opinion in Cardiology. 2011;**26**(3):245-255

[10] Klotz S, Jan Danser AH, Burkhoff D. Impact of left ventricular assist device (LVAD) support on the cardiac reverse remodeling process. Progress in Biophysics and Molecular Biology. 2008;**97**(2-3):479-496

[11] Mann DL, Barger PM, Burkhoff D. Myocardial recovery and the failing heart: Myth, magic, or molecular target? Journal of the American College of Cardiology. 2012;**60**(24):2465-2472

[12] Ambardekar AV, Buttrick PM. Reverse remodeling with left ventricular assist devices: A review of clinical, cellular, and molecular effects. Circulation. Heart Failure. 2011;**4**(2):224-233

[13] Birks EJ. Molecular changes after left ventricular assist device support for heart failure. Circulation Research. 2013;**113**(6):777-791

[14] Hall JL et al. Clinical, molecular, and genomic changes in response to a left ventricular assist device. Journal of the American College of Cardiology. 2011;**57**(6):641-652

[15] Terracciano CM et al. Clinical recovery from end-stage heart failure using left-ventricular assist device and pharmacological therapy correlates with increased sarcoplasmic reticulum calcium content but not with regression of cellular hypertrophy. Circulation. 2004;**109**(19):2263-2265

[16] Birks EJ et al. Gene profiling changes in cytoskeletal proteins during clinical

recovery after left ventricular-assist device support. Circulation. 2005;**112**(9 Suppl):I57-I64

[17] Klotz S et al. Mechanical unloading during left ventricular assist device support increases left ventricular collagen cross-linking and myocardial stiffness. Circulation. 2005;**112**(3):364-374

[18] Jiang M et al. Mitochondrial metabolism in myocardial Remodeling and mechanical unloading: Implications for ischemic heart disease. Frontiers in Cardiovascular Medicine. 2021;**8**:789267

[19] Bhavsar PK et al. Clenbuterol induces cardiac myocyte hypertrophy via paracrine signalling and fibroblast-derived IGF-1. Journal of Cardiovascular Translational Research. 2010;**3**(6):688-695

[20] Hall JL et al. Molecular signature of recovery following combination left ventricular assist device (LVAD) support and pharmacologic therapy. European Heart Journal. 2007;**28**(5):613-627

[21] Burkhoff D et al. Reverse Remodeling with left ventricular assist devices. Circulation Research. 2021;**128**(10):1594-1612

[22] Miyagawa S et al. Building a bridge to recovery: The pathophysiology of LVAD-induced reverse modeling in heart failure. Surgery Today. 2016;**46**(2):149-154

[23] McDonagh TA et al. 2021 ESC guidelines for the diagnosis and treatment of acute and chronic heart failure. European Heart Journal. 2021;**42**(36):3599-3726

[24] Sciaccaluga C et al. Biomarkers in patients with left ventricular assist device: An insight on current evidence. Biomolecules. 2022;**12**(2):334

[25] Wohlschlaeger J et al. Reverse remodeling following insertion of left ventricular assist devices (LVAD): A review of the morphological and molecular changes. Cardiovascular Research. 2005;**68**(3):376-386

[26] Abassi Z et al. Implications of the natriuretic peptide system in the pathogenesis of heart failure: Diagnostic and therapeutic importance. Pharmacology & Therapeutics. 2004;**102**(3):223-241

[27] Sodian R et al. Decreased plasma concentration of brain natriuretic peptide as a potential indicator of cardiac recovery in patients supported by mechanical circulatory assist systems. Journal of the American College of Cardiology. 2001;**38**(7):1942-1949

[28] Bruggink AH et al. Brain natriuretic peptide is produced both by cardiomyocytes and cells infiltrating the heart in patients with severe heart failure supported by a left ventricular assist device. The Journal of Heart and Lung Transplantation. 2006;**25**(2):174-180

[29] Kuhn M et al. Left ventricular assist device support reverses altered cardiac expression and function of natriuretic peptides and receptors in end-stage heart failure. Cardiovascular Research. 2004;**64**(2):308-314

[30] Angelone T, Mazza R, Cerra MC. Chromogranin-a: A multifaceted cardiovascular role in health and disease. Current Medicinal Chemistry. 2012;**19**(24):4042-4050

[31] Pieroni M et al. Myocardial production of chromogranin a in human heart: A new regulatory peptide

of cardiac function. European Heart Journal. 2007;**28**(9):1117-1127

[32] Wohlschlaeger J et al. Decreased myocardial chromogranin a expression and colocalization with brain natriuretic peptide during reverse cardiac remodeling after ventricular unloading. The Journal of Heart and Lung Transplantation. 2008;**27**(4):442-449

[33] Milting H et al. The time course of natriuretic hormones as plasma markers of myocardial recovery in heart transplant candidates during ventricular assist device support reveals differences among device types. The Journal of Heart and Lung Transplantation. 2001;**20**(9):949-955

[34] Wong DT et al. Effectiveness of serial increases in amino-terminal pro-B-type natriuretic peptide levels to indicate the need for mechanical circulatory support in children with acute decompensated heart failure. The American Journal of Cardiology. 2011;**107**(4):573-578

[35] Mohapatra B et al. Short-term mechanical unloading and reverse remodeling of failing hearts in children. The Journal of Heart and Lung Transplantation. 2010;**29**(1):98-104

[36] Schmieder RE et al. Renin-angiotensin system and cardiovascular risk. Lancet. 2007;**369**(9568):1208-1219

[37] Chaggar PS et al. Neuroendocrine effects on the heart and targets for therapeutic manipulation in heart failure. Cardiovascular Therapeutics. 2009;**27**(3):187-193

[38] Messmann R et al. Alterations of the renin angiotensin system in human end-stage heart failure before and after mechanical cardiac unloading by LVAD support. Molecular and Cellular Biochemistry. 2020;**472**(1-2):79-94

[39] Grupper A et al. Effect of Neurohormonal blockade drug therapy on outcomes and left ventricular function and structure after left ventricular assist device implantation. The American Journal of Cardiology. 2016;**117**(11):1765-1770

[40] Klotz S et al. The impact of angiotensin-converting enzyme inhibitor therapy on the extracellular collagen matrix during left ventricular assist device support in patients with end-stage heart failure. Journal of the American College of Cardiology. 2007;**49**(11):1166-1174

[41] Brinkley DM Jr et al. Impact of renin-angiotensin-aldosterone system inhibition on morbidity and mortality during long-term continuous-flow left ventricular assist device support: An IMACS report. The Journal of Heart and Lung Transplantation. 2021;**40**(12):1605-1613

[42] Radley G et al. The inflammatory response to ventricular assist devices. Frontiers in Immunology. 2018;**9**:2651

[43] Torre-Amione G et al. Decreased expression of tumor necrosis factor-alpha in failing human myocardium after mechanical circulatory support : A potential mechanism for cardiac recovery. Circulation. 1999;**100**(11):1189-1193

[44] Bryant D et al. Cardiac failure in transgenic mice with myocardial expression of tumor necrosis factor-alpha. Circulation. 1998;**97**(14):1375-1381

[45] Torre-Amione G et al. Proinflammatory cytokine levels in patients with depressed left ventricular ejection fraction: A report from the studies of left ventricular dysfunction (SOLVD). Journal of

the American College of Cardiology. 1996;**27**(5):1201-1206

[46] Birks EJ et al. Quantitative myocardial cytokine expression and activation of the apoptotic pathway in patients who require left ventricular assist devices. Circulation. 2001;**104**(12 Suppl 1):I233-I240

[47] Kagi JH, Schaffer A. Biochemistry of metallothionein. Biochemistry. 1988;**27**(23):8509-8515

[48] Jin T, Lu J, Nordberg M. Toxicokinetics and biochemistry of cadmium with special emphasis on the role of metallothionein. Neurotoxicology. 1998;**19**(4-5):529-535

[49] Baba HA et al. Metallothionein: Localization in human transplant endomyocardium, relation to cytokines and allograft function. The Journal of Heart and Lung Transplantation. 1999;**18**(10):963-971

[50] Baba HA et al. Reversal of metallothionein expression is different throughout the human myocardium after prolonged left-ventricular mechanical support. The Journal of Heart and Lung Transplantation. 2000;**19**(7):668-674

[51] Batra J et al. C-reactive protein levels predict outcomes in continuous-flow left ventricular assist device patients: An INTERMACS analysis. ASAIO Journal. 2021;**67**(8):884-890

[52] Syeda T et al. Pre- and post-operative values of serum CRP in patients undergoing surgery for brain tumour. The Journal of the Pakistan Medical Association. 2014;**64**(3):271-274

[53] Ahmad T et al. Effects of left ventricular assist device support on biomarkers of cardiovascular stress, fibrosis, fluid homeostasis, inflammation, and renal injury. JACC Heart Fail. 2015;**3**(1):30-39

[54] Niazy N et al. Altered mRNA expression of Interleukin-1 receptors in myocardial tissue of patients with left ventricular assist device support. Journal of Clinical Medicine. 2021;**10**(21):4856

[55] Kotsiou OS, Gourgoulianis KI, Zarogiannis SG. IL-33/ST2 Axis in organ fibrosis. Frontiers in Immunology. 2018;**9**:2432

[56] Millar NL et al. Wounds that heal and wounds that don't - the role of the IL-33/ST2 pathway in tissue repair and tumorigenesis. Seminars in Cell & Developmental Biology. 2017;**61**:41-50

[57] Tseng CCS et al. The Interleukin-33/ST2 pathway is expressed in the failing human heart and associated with pro-fibrotic Remodeling of the myocardium. Journal of Cardiovascular Translational Research. 2018;**11**(1):15-21

[58] Tseng CCS et al. Soluble ST2 in end-stage heart failure, before and after support with a left ventricular assist device. European Journal of Clinical Investigation. 2018;**48**(3):e12886

[59] Caselli C et al. IL-33/ST2 pathway and classical cytokines in end-stage heart failure patients submitted to left ventricular assist device support: A paradoxic role for inflammatory mediators? Mediators of Inflammation. 2013;**2013**:498703

[60] Cabiati M et al. Transcriptional evaluation of relaxin and endothelin-1 axis in heart failure patients: First evidence of its involvement during left ventricular assist device support. International Journal of Cardiology. 2020;**306**:109-115

[61] Coromilas E et al. Dynamics and prognostic role of galectin-3 in patients

with advanced heart failure, during left ventricular assist device support and following heart transplantation. BMC Cardiovascular Disorders. 2016;**16**:138

[62] Lok SI et al. Myocardial fibrosis and pro-fibrotic markers in end-stage heart failure patients during continuous-flow left ventricular assist device support. European Journal of Cardio-Thoracic Surgery. 2015;**48**(3):407-415

[63] Banerjee I et al. Determination of cell types and numbers during cardiac development in the neonatal and adult rat and mouse. American Journal of Physiology. Heart and Circulatory Physiology. 2007;**293**(3):H1883-H1891

[64] Heineke J, Molkentin JD. Regulation of cardiac hypertrophy by intracellular signalling pathways. Nature Reviews. Molecular Cell Biology. 2006;**7**(8):589-600

[65] Harvey PA, Leinwand LA. The cell biology of disease: Cellular mechanisms of cardiomyopathy. The Journal of Cell Biology. 2011;**194**(3):355-365

[66] Shen S, Sewanan LR, Campbell SG. Evidence for synergy between sarcomeres and fibroblasts in an in vitro model of myocardial reverse remodeling. Journal of Molecular and Cellular Cardiology. 2021;**158**:11-25

[67] Ma ZG et al. Cardiac fibrosis: New insights into the pathogenesis. International Journal of Biological Sciences. 2018;**14**(12):1645-1657

[68] Nielsen SH et al. Understanding cardiac extracellular matrix remodeling to develop biomarkers of myocardial infarction outcomes. Matrix Biology. 2019;**75-76**:43-57

[69] Bishop JE et al. Enhanced deposition of predominantly type I collagen in myocardial disease. Journal of Molecular and Cellular Cardiology. 1990;**22**(10):1157-1165

[70] Nikolov A, Popovski N. Extracellular matrix in heart disease: Focus on circulating collagen type I and III derived peptides as biomarkers of myocardial fibrosis and their potential in the prognosis of heart failure: A concise review. Metabolites. 2022;**12**(4):297

[71] Bruckner BA et al. Regression of fibrosis and hypertrophy in failing myocardium following mechanical circulatory support. The Journal of Heart and Lung Transplantation. 2001;**20**(4):457-464

[72] Barton PJ et al. Myocardial insulin-like growth factor-I gene expression during recovery from heart failure after combined left ventricular assist device and clenbuterol therapy. Circulation. 2005;**112**(9 Suppl):I46-I50

[73] Brew K, Nagase H. The tissue inhibitors of metalloproteinases (TIMPs): An ancient family with structural and functional diversity. Biochimica et Biophysica Acta. 2010;**1803**(1):55-71

[74] Barton PJ et al. Increased expression of extracellular matrix regulators TIMP1 and MMP1 in deteriorating heart failure. The Journal of Heart and Lung Transplantation. 2003;**22**(7):738-744

[75] Felkin LE et al. A quantitative gene expression profile of matrix metalloproteinases (MMPS) and their inhibitors (TIMPS) in the myocardium of patients with deteriorating heart failure requiring left ventricular assist device support. The Journal of Heart and Lung Transplantation. 2006;**25**(12):1413-1419

[76] Bruggink AH et al. Type IV collagen degradation in the myocardial

basement membrane after unloading of the failing heart by a left ventricular assist device. Laboratory Investigation. 2007;**87**(11):1125-1137

[77] Butler CR, Jugdutt BI. The paradox of left ventricular assist device unloading and myocardial recovery in end-stage dilated cardiomyopathy: Implications for heart failure in the elderly. Heart Failure Reviews. 2012;**17**(4-5):615-633

[78] Wang G et al. Role of endothelial and mesenchymal cell transitions in heart failure and recovery thereafter. Frontiers in Genetics. 2020;**11**:609262

[79] Hall JL et al. Genomic profiling of the human heart before and after mechanical support with a ventricular assist device reveals alterations in vascular signaling networks. Physiological Genomics. 2004;**17**(3):283-291

[80] Drakos SG et al. Impact of mechanical unloading on microvasculature and associated central remodeling features of the failing human heart. Journal of the American College of Cardiology. 2010;**56**(5):382-391

[81] Zafeiridis A et al. Regression of cellular hypertrophy after left ventricular assist device support. Circulation. 1998;**98**(7):656-662

[82] Diakos NA et al. Myocardial atrophy and chronic mechanical unloading of the failing human heart: Implications for cardiac assist device-induced myocardial recovery. Journal of the American College of Cardiology. 2014;**64**(15):1602-1612

[83] Breitbart A et al. Myostatin from the heart: Local and systemic actions in cardiac failure and muscle wasting. American Journal of Physiology. Heart and Circulatory Physiology. 2011;**300**(6):H1973-H1982

[84] George I et al. Myostatin activation in patients with advanced heart failure and after mechanical unloading. European Journal of Heart Failure. 2010;**12**(5):444-453

[85] Gordon JW, Shaw JA, Kirshenbaum LA. Multiple facets of NF-kappaB in the heart: To be or not to NF-kappaB. Circulation Research. 2011;**108**(9):1122-1132

[86] Zelarayan L et al. NF-kappaB activation is required for adaptive cardiac hypertrophy. Cardiovascular Research. 2009;**84**(3):416-424

[87] Hamid T et al. Divergent tumor necrosis factor receptor-related remodeling responses in heart failure: Role of nuclear factor-kappaB and inflammatory activation. Circulation. 2009;**119**(10):1386-1397

[88] Grabellus F et al. Reversible activation of nuclear factor-kappaB in human end-stage heart failure after left ventricular mechanical support. Cardiovascular Research. 2002;**53**(1):124-130

[89] Baba HA et al. Dynamic regulation of MEK/Erks and Akt/GSK-3beta in human end-stage heart failure after left ventricular mechanical support: Myocardial mechanotransduction-sensitivity as a possible molecular mechanism. Cardiovascular Research. 2003;**59**(2):390-399

[90] Razeghi P et al. Mechanical unloading of the failing human heart fails to activate the protein kinase B/Akt/glycogen synthase kinase-3beta survival pathway. Cardiology. 2003;**100**(1):17-22

[91] Flesch M et al. Differential regulation of mitogen-activated protein kinases in the failing human heart in response

to mechanical unloading. Circulation. 2001;**104**(19):2273-2276

[92] Stawowy P et al. Increased myocardial expression of osteopontin in patients with advanced heart failure. European Journal of Heart Failure. 2002;**4**(2):139-146

[93] Schipper ME et al. Osteopontin: A potential biomarker for heart failure and reverse remodeling after left ventricular assist device support. The Journal of Heart and Lung Transplantation. 2011;**30**(7):805-810

[94] Prescimone T et al. Cardiac molecular markers of programmed cell death are activated in end-stage heart failure patients supported by left ventricular assist device. Cardiovascular Pathology. 2014;**23**(5):272-282

[95] Prescimone T et al. Caspase-1 transcripts in failing human heart after mechanical unloading. Cardiovascular Pathology. 2015;**24**(1):11-18

[96] Francis GS et al. Apoptosis, Bcl-2, and proliferating cell nuclear antigen in the failing human heart: Observations made after implantation of left ventricular assist device. Journal of Cardiac Failure. 1999;**5**(4):308-315

[97] Kassiotis C et al. Markers of autophagy are downregulated in failing human heart after mechanical unloading. Circulation. 2009;**120**(11 Suppl):S191-S197

[98] Bedi MS et al. Myocardial Fas and cytokine expression in end-stage heart failure: Impact of LVAD support. Clinical and Translational Science. 2008;**1**(3):245-248

[99] Purevjav E et al. Myocardial Fas ligand expression increases susceptibility to AZT-induced cardiomyopathy. Cardiovascular Toxicology. 2007;**7**(4):255-263

[100] Bartling B et al. Myocardial gene expression of regulators of myocyte apoptosis and myocyte calcium homeostasis during hemodynamic unloading by ventricular assist devices in patients with end-stage heart failure. Circulation. 1999;**100**(19 Suppl):216-223

[101] Castillero E et al. Structural and functional cardiac profile after prolonged duration of mechanical unloading: Potential implications for myocardial recovery. American Journal of Physiology. Heart and Circulatory Physiology. 2018;**315**(5):H1463-H1476

[102] de Jonge N et al. Cardiomyocyte death in patients with end-stage heart failure before and after support with a left ventricular assist device: Low incidence of apoptosis despite ubiquitous mediators. The Journal of Heart and Lung Transplantation. 2003;**22**(9):1028-1036

[103] Ron D, Walter P. Signal integration in the endoplasmic reticulum unfolded protein response. Nature Reviews. Molecular Cell Biology. 2007;**8**(7):519-529

[104] Castillero E et al. Attenuation of the unfolded protein response and endoplasmic reticulum stress after mechanical unloading in dilated cardiomyopathy. American Journal of Physiology. Heart and Circulatory Physiology. 2015;**309**(3):H459-H470

[105] Yuan X, Braun T. Multimodal regulation of cardiac myocyte proliferation. Circulation Research. 2017;**121**(3):293-309

[106] Sandritter W, Adler CP. Polyploidization of heart muscle nuclei as a prerequisite for heart growth

and numerical hyperplasia in heart hypertrophy. Recent Advances in Studies on Cardiac Structure and Metabolism. 1976;**12**:115-127

[107] Gonzalez-Rosa JM et al. Myocardial Polyploidization creates a barrier to heart regeneration in zebrafish. Developmental Cell. 2018;**44**(4):433-446 e7

[108] Wohlschlaeger J et al. Hemodynamic support by left ventricular assist devices reduces cardiomyocyte DNA content in the failing human heart. Circulation. 2010;**121**(8):989-996

[109] Canseco DC et al. Human ventricular unloading induces cardiomyocyte proliferation. Journal of the American College of Cardiology. 2015;**65**(9):892-900

[110] Kim GH, Uriel N, Burkhoff D. Reverse remodelling and myocardial recovery in heart failure. Nature Reviews. Cardiology. 2018;**15**(2):83-96

[111] Margulies KB et al. Mixed messages: Transcription patterns in failing and recovering human myocardium. Circulation Research. 2005;**96**(5):592-599

[112] Cullen ME et al. Myocardial expression of the arginine:Glycine amidinotransferase gene is elevated in heart failure and normalized after recovery: Potential implications for local creatine synthesis. Circulation. 2006;**114**(1 Suppl):I16-I20

[113] Weia BC, Adachi I, Jacot JG. Clinical and molecular comparison of Pediatric and adult reverse Remodeling with ventricular assist devices. Artificial Organs. 2015;**39**(8):691-700

[114] Sugawara K et al. Structure and functional roles of Epac2 (Rapgef4). Gene. 2016;**575**(2 Pt 3):577-583

[115] Saunders MA, Liang H, Li WH. Human polymorphism at microRNAs and microRNA target sites. Proceedings of the National Academy of Sciences of the United States of America. 2007;**104**(9):3300-3305

[116] Peterlin A et al. The role of microRNAs in heart failure: A systematic review. Frontiers in Cardiovascular Medicine. 2020;**7**:161

[117] Matkovich SJ et al. Reciprocal regulation of myocardial microRNAs and messenger RNA in human cardiomyopathy and reversal of the microRNA signature by biomechanical support. Circulation. 2009;**119**(9):1263-1271

[118] Ragusa R et al. Epigenetic regulation of cardiac troponin genes in Pediatric patients with heart failure supported by ventricular assist device. Biomedicine. 2021;**9**(10):1409

[119] Ragusa R et al. Variations of circulating miRNA in paediatric patients with heart failure supported with ventricular assist device: A pilot study. Scientific Reports. 2020;**10**(1):5905

[120] Bristow MR et al. Decreased catecholamine sensitivity and beta-adrenergic-receptor density in failing human hearts. The New England Journal of Medicine. 1982;**307**(4):205-211

[121] Ungerer M et al. Altered expression of beta-adrenergic receptor kinase and beta 1-adrenergic receptors in the failing human heart. Circulation. 1993;**87**(2):454-463

[122] Pandalai PK et al. Restoration of myocardial beta-adrenergic receptor signaling after left ventricular assist device support. The Journal of Thoracic and Cardiovascular Surgery. 2006;**131**(5):975-980

[123] Ogletree-Hughes ML et al. Mechanical unloading restores beta-adrenergic responsiveness and reverses receptor downregulation in the failing human heart. Circulation. 2001;**104**(8):881-886

[124] Akhter SA et al. Reversal of impaired myocardial beta-adrenergic receptor signaling by continuous-flow left ventricular assist device support. The Journal of Heart and Lung Transplantation. 2010;**29**(6):603-609

[125] Medina E et al. Molecular changes in children with heart failure undergoing left ventricular assist device therapy. The Journal of Pediatrics. 2017;**182**:184-189 e1

[126] Francis SH, Corbin JD. Cyclic nucleotide-dependent protein kinases: Intracellular receptors for cAMP and cGMP action. Critical Reviews in Clinical Laboratory Sciences. 1999;**36**(4):275-328

[127] Persoon S et al. Cardiac unloading by LVAD support differentially influences components of the cGMP-PKG signaling pathway in ischemic and dilated cardiomyopathy. Heart and Vessels. 2018;**33**(8):948-957

[128] Grosman-Rimon L et al. Increased cyclic guanosine monophosphate levels and continuous-flow left-ventricular assist devices: Implications for gastrointestinal bleeding. The Journal of Thoracic and Cardiovascular Surgery. 2016;**151**(1):219-227

[129] Stetson SJ et al. Improved myocardial structure following LVAD support: Effect of unloading on dystrophin expression. The Journal of Heart and Lung Transplantation. 2001;**20**(2):240

[130] de Jonge N et al. Left ventricular assist device in end-stage heart failure: Persistence of structural myocyte damage after unloading. An immunohistochemical analysis of the contractile myofilaments. Journal of the American College of Cardiology. 2002;**39**(6):963-969

[131] Tennyson CN, Klamut HJ, Worton RG. The human dystrophin gene requires 16 hours to be transcribed and is cotranscriptionally spliced. Nature Genetics. 1995;**9**(2):184-190

[132] Hoffman EP, Brown RH Jr, Kunkel LM. Dystrophin: The protein product of the Duchenne muscular dystrophy locus. Cell. 1987;**51**(6):919-928

[133] Le Rumeur E. Dystrophin and the two related genetic diseases, Duchenne and Becker muscular dystrophies. Bosnian Journal of Basic Medical Sciences. 2015;**15**(3):14-20

[134] Towbin JA et al. X-linked dilated cardiomyopathy. Molecular genetic evidence of linkage to the Duchenne muscular dystrophy (dystrophin) gene at the Xp21 locus. Circulation. 1993;**87**(6):1854-1865

[135] Vatta M et al. Molecular remodelling of dystrophin in patients with end-stage cardiomyopathies and reversal in patients on assistance-device therapy. Lancet. 2002;**359**(9310):936-941

[136] Berridge MJ. Calcium signalling remodelling and disease. Biochemical Society Transactions. 2012;**40**(2):297-309

[137] Smith GL, Eisner DA. Calcium buffering in the heart in health and disease. Circulation. 2019;**139**(20):2358-2371

[138] Mishra S et al. Molecular mechanisms of reduced sarcoplasmic reticulum Ca(2+) uptake in human failing left ventricular myocardium.

The Journal of Heart and Lung Transplantation. 2002;**21**(3):366-373

[139] Schillinger W et al. Influence of SR Ca(2+)-ATPase and Na(+)-Ca(2+)-exchanger on the force-frequency relation. Basic Research in Cardiology. 1998;**93**(Suppl. 1):38-45

[140] Pieske B et al. Ca2+ handling and sarcoplasmic reticulum Ca2+ content in isolated failing and nonfailing human myocardium. Circulation Research. 1999;**85**(1):38-46

[141] Chaudhary KW et al. Altered myocardial Ca2+ cycling after left ventricular assist device support in the failing human heart. Journal of the American College of Cardiology. 2004;**44**(4):837-845

[142] Madigan JD et al. Time course of reverse remodeling of the left ventricle during support with a left ventricular assist device. The Journal of Thoracic and Cardiovascular Surgery. 2001;**121**(5):902-908

[143] Ogletree ML et al. Duration of left ventricular assist device support: Effects on abnormal calcium cycling and functional recovery in the failing human heart. The Journal of Heart and Lung Transplantation. 2010;**29**(5):554-561

[144] Heerdt PM et al. Chronic unloading by left ventricular assist device reverses contractile dysfunction and alters gene expression in end-stage heart failure. Circulation. 2000;**102**(22):2713-2719

[145] Huss JM, Kelly DP. Mitochondrial energy metabolism in heart failure: A question of balance. The Journal of Clinical Investigation. 2005;**115**(3):547-555

[146] Cluntun AA et al. The pyruvate-lactate axis modulates cardiac hypertrophy and heart failure. Cell Metabolism. 2021;**33**(3):629-648 e10

[147] Jaswal JS et al. Targeting fatty acid and carbohydrate oxidation--a novel therapeutic intervention in the ischemic and failing heart. Biochimica et Biophysica Acta. 2011;**1813**(7):1333-1350

[148] Diakos NA et al. Evidence of glycolysis up-regulation and pyruvate mitochondrial oxidation mismatch during mechanical unloading of the failing human heart: Implications for cardiac reloading and conditioning. JACC Basic to Translational Science. 2016;**1**(6):432-444

[149] Chokshi A et al. Ventricular assist device implantation corrects myocardial lipotoxicity, reverses insulin resistance, and normalizes cardiac metabolism in patients with advanced heart failure. Circulation. 2012;**125**(23):2844-2853

[150] Ahmad T et al. Prognostic implications of long-chain Acylcarnitines in heart failure and reversibility with mechanical circulatory support. Journal of the American College of Cardiology. 2016;**67**(3):291-299

[151] Badolia R et al. The role of nonglycolytic glucose metabolism in myocardial recovery upon mechanical unloading and circulatory support in chronic heart failure. Circulation. 2020;**142**(3):259-274

[152] Lee SH et al. Improvement of myocardial mitochondrial function after hemodynamic support with left ventricular assist devices in patients with heart failure. The Journal of Thoracic and Cardiovascular Surgery. 1998;**116**(2):344-349

[153] Scheiber D et al. Reduced myocardial mitochondrial ROS production in mechanically

unloaded hearts. Journal of Cardiovascular Translational Research. 2019;**12**(2):107-115

[154] Shahinian JH et al. Impact of left ventricular assist device therapy on the cardiac proteome and metabolome composition in ischemic cardiomyopathy. Artificial Organs. 2020;**44**(3):257-267

[155] Boyman L, Karbowski M, Lederer WJ. Regulation of mitochondrial ATP production: Ca(2+) Signaling and quality control. Trends in Molecular Medicine. 2020;**26**(1):21-39

[156] McCormack JG, Halestrap AP, Denton RM. Role of calcium ions in regulation of mammalian intramitochondrial metabolism. Physiological Reviews. 1990;**70**(2):391-425

[157] Ramachandra CJA et al. Mitochondria in acute myocardial infarction and cardioprotection. eBioMedicine. 2020;**57**:102884

[158] Kohlhaas M, Maack C. Adverse bioenergetic consequences of Na+-Ca2+ exchanger-mediated Ca2+ influx in cardiac myocytes. Circulation. 2010;**122**(22):2273-2280

[159] Dolinsky VW et al. Cardiac mitochondrial energy metabolism in heart failure: Role of cardiolipin and sirtuins. Biochimica et Biophysica Acta. 2016;**1861**(10):1544-1554

[160] Heerdt PM et al. Disease-specific remodeling of cardiac mitochondria after a left ventricular assist device. The Annals of Thoracic Surgery. 2002;**73**(4):1216-1221

[161] D'Amico A et al. Uncovering the cathepsin system in heart failure patients submitted to left ventricular assist device (LVAD) implantation. Journal of Translational Medicine. 2014;**12**:350

[162] Rose BA, Force T, Wang Y. Mitogen-activated protein kinase signaling in the heart: Angels versus demons in a heart-breaking tale. Physiological Reviews. 2010;**90**(4):1507-1546

[163] Communal C, Colucci WS, Singh K. p38 mitogen-activated protein kinase pathway protects adult rat ventricular myocytes against beta -adrenergic receptor-stimulated apoptosis. Evidence for Gi-dependent activation. The Journal of Biological Chemistry. 2000;**275**(25):19395-19400

[164] Wang Y et al. Cardiac muscle cell hypertrophy and apoptosis induced by distinct members of the p38 mitogen-activated protein kinase family. The Journal of Biological Chemistry. 1998;**273**(4):2161-2168

[165] Cook SA, Sugden PH, Clerk A. Activation of c-Jun N-terminal kinases and p38-mitogen-activated protein kinases in human heart failure secondary to ischaemic heart disease. Journal of Molecular and Cellular Cardiology. 1999;**31**(8):1429-1434

[166] Haq S et al. Differential activation of signal transduction pathways in human hearts with hypertrophy versus advanced heart failure. Circulation. 2001;**103**(5):670-677

[167] Gallo S et al. ERK: A key player in the pathophysiology of cardiac hypertrophy. International Journal of Molecular Sciences. 2019;**20**(9):2164

[168] Abeyrathna P, Su Y. The critical role of Akt in cardiovascular function. Vascular Pharmacology. 2015;**74**:38-48

[169] Marinescu KK et al. Left ventricular assist device-induced reverse remodeling: it's not just about myocardial recovery. Expert Review of Medical Devices. 2017;**14**(1):15-26

Section 3

Arrhythmia Management during Mechanical Circulatory Support

Chapter 3

Arrhythmia Management in Pediatric Patients with Ventricular Assist Devices

Karine Guerrier and Ahmad Sami Chaouki

Abstract

Ventricular assist device therapy has emerged as an important approach in the management of advanced heart failure. Atrial and ventricular arrhythmias are commonly encountered in patients with heart failure. Patients requiring ventricular assist devices are at an increased risk of arrhythmia, which may cause symptoms and significant complications. There is recent focus on the prevalence and impact of atrial and ventricular arrhythmias in patients with durable ventricular assist devices. Ventricular arrhythmias in particular have been associated with significant symptoms and worse clinical outcomes. The goal of this chapter is to outline approaches to arrhythmia management in pediatric patients with ventricular assist devices.

Keywords: ventricular arrhythmia, ventricular assist device, supraventricular arrhythmia, mechanical support, pediatric, management

1. Introduction

Heart failure in children is a growing global public health concern. In the United States, approximately 14,000 children are hospitalized for heart failure annually [1]. Symptoms of heart failure may include poor feeding, poor growth, and exercise intolerance. Heart failure in pediatric patients has various etiologies including failing physiology in congenital heart disease, inflammatory disease such as myocarditis, arrhythmia, post chemotherapy exposure, primary cardiomyopathy, and cardiac transplant rejection. Patients with congenital heart disease are at increased risk for developing heart failure secondary to chronic volume overload, elevated atrial and ventricular pressure, inadequate myocardial perfusion, and persistent ventricular dysfunction following surgical intervention. It has been reported that approximately 70% of hospital admissions for pediatric heart failure involve patients with congenital heart disease [1]. The risk for heart failure in congenital heart disease increases with age, with nearly 25% of adult congenital heart disease patients experiencing heart failure by the age of 30 years [2]. The Fontan palliation has been associated with high risk of developing heart failure with independent predictors of single morphological right ventricle, higher right atrial pressure, and evidence of protein-losing enteropathy [3].

 IntechOpen

Heart failure in children is associated with high morbidity and mortality with 20-fold increased risk of death during hospitalization [4, 5]. Noncardiac complications may include sepsis, renal failure, and respiratory failure. Studies have demonstrated that factors associated with increased risk of hospital mortality include acute renal failure and hepatic injury [1]. Early intervention with appropriate medical therapy is important in the management of acute heart failure. In cases where conventional therapies are not sufficient, mechanical circulatory support may be necessary.

Ventricular assist device (VAD) therapy has emerged as an important tool in the management of severe and refractory heart failure. An increasing number of patients are supported by a VAD, improving survival of patients whether used as destination therapy, bridge to transplantation, or bridge to cardiac function recovery. Over 25,000 VADs have been implanted in the United States [6] and the number of devices implanted in pediatric patients has increased over the years [7–9]. Cardiomyopathy, congenital heart disease, and myocarditis are the most frequently encountered underlying conditions in pediatric heart failure patients requiring VAD therapy [10, 11]. As there is increased risk for atrial and ventricular tachyarrhythmias in patients with heart failure, it is not uncommon to encounter these arrhythmias following VAD implantation.

2. Ventricular assist devices

Mechanical circulatory support has become increasingly common in the management of heart failure. The initial objective of VAD therapy was a temporary form of mechanical circulatory support as a bridge to cardiac transplantation. Improved survival with VADs and deficient donor organ supply has since resulted in increased use as destination therapy. In modern practice, VADs are often used as chronic therapy or permanent circulatory support.

Device selection and timing of initiating VAD support are vital in optimizing cardiac function recovery and chance for survival. Anatomic variations secondary to congenital heart disease or surgical interventions pose technical challenges to VAD implantation [12]. Other factors including severe neurologic impairment, chromosomal or congenital anomalies with anticipated poor outcome and significant prematurity or low body weight should be taken into consideration prior to VAD implantation. Patient size, anticipated duration, type of support, and ultimate goal of therapy are important elements in device selection.

The EXCOR © (Berlin Heart) is specifically designed for infants and children, providing mechanical circulatory support via pulsatile membrane pumps. The system offers multiple pump and cannula sizes to accommodate different patient sizes. It is important to avoid mismatch between patient and device size as mismatch has been associated with poor outcome [12]. Unfortunately, early generation VADs utilizing pulsatile flow were characterized by high rates of complications including high incidence of device failure and poor survival. These early devices were preload-dependent and sensitive to changes in cardiac output including those related to arrhythmia. There has been notable improvement in patient survival and reduction in complications with transition to continuous flow VADs [8].

There are two subclassifications of continuous flow VAD design – axial and centrifugal. In general, axial flow is generated by a propeller in a pipe with filling completed by use of negative pressure while a bladed disk spinning in a cavity generates centrifugal flow [13]. The second-generation VAD HeartMate II © (Abbott) provides short or long-term circulatory support for heart failure patients as a continuous flow system that funds via axial flow generated with mechanical bearings. It has a lower incidence of thromboembolic events compared to the first-generation VADs [12, 13]. The HVAD pump (HeartWare Inc) is a continuous-flow device with a centrifugal pump that is attached directly to the inflow cannula. It is smaller than the HeartMate II and, with adjustment in the implantation technique, has demonstrated utility in the pediatric heart failure population [14]. While output from continuous flow VADs is not immediately affected by arrhythmias, there may still be hemodynamic instability from deficient right ventricular support. Third generation VADs, HeartMate 3© (Abbott), generate continuous flow via a centrifugal flow pump utilizing a magnetically levitated rotor. The CentriMag/PediMag© (Abbott) is a centrifugal pump that is used for temporary support. The presence of arrhythmia may lead to a reduction in preload and subsequent decrease in device flow [15].

In select patients with severe biventricular systolic dysfunction, complete replacement of the ventricles may be warranted. This is achieved with temporary total artificial hearts (TAH, Syncardia). These devices provide global circulatory support through a pneumatic pulsatile pump with an external portable drive. The temporary total artificial heart is traditionally utilized as a bridge to transplantation.

The use of VADs in pediatric heart failure patients has increased in the past decade [7, 9, 16]. While the use of pulsatile-flow and continuous flow devices in pediatric patients have each increased over time, pulsatile-flow devices were more frequently utilized in younger, smaller patients and those with congenital heart disease [16]. In this population, the majority of VADs were implanted as bridge to transplant.

3. Pathophysiology of arrhythmias encountered in patients with ventricular assist devices

Pediatric patients with decompensated heart failure are at increased risk for tachyarrhythmias. Patients requiring VAD therapy are at high risk for atrial and ventricular arrhythmias. In one cohort, over 70% of children with VADs experienced an arrhythmia with nearly 20% developing new arrhythmia while on VAD therapy [11]. Ventricular tachycardia is consistently the most common arrhythmia reported post VAD implantation, with documentation of monomorphic and polymorphic ventricular tachycardia. The presence of ventricular arrhythmia prior to VAD therapy has been found to be predictive of ventricular arrhythmia post VAD implantation [17]. More than half of pediatric patients with arrhythmia prior to VAD therapy continue to experience arrhythmia while on VAD [11].

One main mechanism by which heart failure increases the risk of atrial fibrillation is through increased left atrial pressures [18]. Anisotropy and reduced atrial conduction velocity develop from scar secondary to the chronic increased left atrial pressure, promoting atrial tachyarrhythmia. Structural remodeling, atrial myopathy, and maladaptive gene expression are other mechanisms by which heart failure can facilitate the development of atrial fibrillation. Heart failure results in a proinflammatory state that leads to structural remodeling mediated by diffuse fibrosis, the consequence of which includes electrophysiologic heterogeneity and slowed conduction [19]. Associated left ventricular diastolic dysfunction transfers increased left ventricular filling pressure to the left atrium. Prolonged elevated left atrial pressure can result in dispersion of refractoriness. Studies have demonstrated prolongation in atrial refractoriness, P-wave duration, and conduction time in patients with atrial fibrillation [20]. Increased left atrial pressure results in decrease in cardiac calcium ion channels, leading to calcium overload, increased diastolic calcium lead, and prolonged action potential duration. Increased calcium content has been demonstrated to portend afterdepolarizations from the pulmonary veins that serve as triggers for atrial fibrillation [21, 22].

There are several factors related to the underlying heart failure that may stimulate development of ventricular arrhythmia. Ventricular dysfunction has been found to be an independent risk factor for arrhythmia associated with VAD therapy [11, 23]. This is not unexpected as severe ventricular dysfunction itself can promote arrhythmia. The development of chamber enlargement, myocardial scar, and subendocardial ischemia can result in myocardial injury and become arrhythmogenic. Focal areas of scar result in a heterogenous area of healthy and infarcted myocardium with different conduction properties and refractoriness in close proximity [24]. This leads to anisotropy and areas of slow conduction, which is prime for reentry. Neurohormonal activation, enhanced catecholamines, electrolyte abnormalities, and altered calcium handling can also contribute to an environment prone to arrhythmia.

VAD implantation has been associated with electrophysiologic changes. Prolongation of the QT and corrected QT interval have been observed post VAD implantation and associated with tachyarrhythmia [25, 26]. Changes in channel regulation including upregulation of the Na^+/Ca^{2+} exchange and downregulation of the voltage-gated K^+ channel, may contribute to increase in action potential duration and development of delayed afterdepolarizations [27]. The VAD implantation process and presence of the device itself can prompt arrhythmia. Apical scar at the site of VAD inflow cannula insertion can contribute to reentrant ventricular tachyarrhythmias. Suction events where the VAD inflow cannula engages the ventricular wall result in decreased device output, reducing cardiac function support and increasing the risk for ventricular arrhythmia [28]. High VAD pump speed, VAD inflow cannula position, and low patient intravascular volume are contributing factors that increase the risk of suction events [13].

4. Arrhythmias encountered in patients with ventricular assist devices

4.1 Atrial tachyarrhythmia

Atrial arrhythmias are common on patients with heart failure. Atrial fibrillation is the most frequently encountered atrial arrhythmia. However, ectopic atrial tachycardia and atrial flutter are seen as well. Persistent atrial flutter can result in loss of AV synchrony and impaired ventricular filling. In certain patients with left VADs, atrial arrhythmias, particularly atrial flutter with rapid ventricular response, have been associated with hemodynamic compromise secondary to decompensated right heart failure [29, 30]. Improvement in right heart failure has been demonstrated after catheter ablation of the atrial flutter [29].

The pathophysiology of heart failure results in structural changes and electrical remodeling that encourage the development of atrial fibrillation. The frequency of atrial fibrillation increases with heart failure severity, reaching approximately 50% of patients with New York Heart Association (NYHA) Class IV classification [31]. In adult patients, atrial fibrillation may be encountered in over 40% of patients on VAD therapy [32]. There are conflicting results regarding the risk of thromboembolic events patients with atrial arrhythmia on VAD therapy; however, the presence of atrial fibrillation prior to VAD therapy has been shown to predict the occurrence of ventricular arrhythmia after VAD implantation [23].

It has been demonstrated that pediatric patients undergoing VAD therapy for cardiomyopathy or myocarditis have an increased risk of developing arrhythmia [10]. In a cohort of pediatric patients with VAD, 38% experienced an atrial arrhythmia [11]. The majority of the tachyarrhythmia episodes were non-sustained with a median rate of 150 bpm. There was no correlation between presence of arrhythmia and mortality [11]. In pediatric patients with VAD for primary diagnosis of arrhythmia, it has been demonstrated that nearly 70% have supraventricular tachycardia, of which nearly 40% are ectopic atrial tachycardia or atrial flutter [33].

4.2 Ventricular tachyarrhythmia

Before discussing the risks of ventricular arrhythmias in the context of pediatric VAD use, it is important to recognize the risks of these arrhythmias in patients with heart failure in general. Regardless of whether the reason for heart failure is secondary to cardiomyopathy or congenital heart disease, risks have been well described [24, 34]. Guidelines and consensus statements include recommendations for management, including the use of anti-arrhythmics as well as indications for implantation of implantable cardioverter-defibrillators (ICDs) [35, 36]. For this reason, many patients who present for VAD implant are already receiving anti-arrhythmics, have ICDs, or both. In fact, there are a handful of pediatric patients who have received VADs specifically for intractable ventricular arrhythmias [33, 37].

Early in the era of adult VAD use, it became clear that there was an association of new onset monomorphic ventricular tachycardia in the months following implant [38]. While the majority of arrhythmias tend to occur during the initial hospitalization at implant, later onset arrhythmias have also been documented [17]. In addition, given that most patients have significant heart failure, many will already have primary or secondary prevention ICDs with a history of ventricular arrhythmias [39]. Pediatric arrhythmia data in VADs are quite scarce. A 2015 study found over half of patients in a single center study developed ventricular arrhythmias [11]. A more recently published single center study found that patients with cardiomyopathy and myocarditis were more likely to have non-sustained and sustained ventricular tachycardia than those with congenital heart disease [10]. Additionally, those who had less left ventricular decompression were at a higher risk for having ventricular arrhythmias. Arrhythmia presence prior to VAD implant was associated with increased risk of ventricular arrhythmias and antiarrhythmic therapy was associated with decreased risk.

While isolated ventricular ectopy and often non-sustained ventricular tachycardia do not require significant intervention in patients with heart failure, once a VAD is implanted these will likely become even less hemodynamically significant given the additional support [40]. With more sustained arrhythmias, one would expect decreased flows given the loss of right ventricular contribution to cardiac output and if sustained enough, right ventricular failure. For this reason, those patients who receive VAD support specifically for intractable arrhythmias often are given biventricular support [41].

5. Management of Arrhythmias Encountered in patients with ventricular assist devices

It is important to note the potential for reversible causes of arrhythmia in pediatric patients with VAD. Electrolyte derangement, consequences of comorbidities, and drug–drug interactions with electrophysiologic effects should be considered. The identification of reversible causes of atrial or ventricular arrhythmia may allow for management with conventional therapies. Limitation of known QT-prolonging medications and proarrhythmic agents is prudent.

Suction events where the VAD inflow cannula interacts with the ventricular wall can result in ventricular arrhythmia [28]. These events may be avoided by reducing high VAD pump speed and avoiding intravascular volume depletion. Recurrent suction events associated with ventricular arrhythmia may require fluid supplementation.

Studies have demonstrated that some adult patients with continuous-flow VAD remain hemodynamically stable while in ventricular tachyarrhythmia including ventricular fibrillation [40, 42–44]. While patients were symptomatic, there was no evidence of end-organ dysfunction as a result of the ventricular arrhythmia. After restoration of sinus rhythm, there was no recurrence of the ventricular arrhythmia [42]. This suggests that there can be hemodynamic stability with left VAD support during episodes of ventricular arrhythmia. However, prolonged ventricular fibrillation can result in right ventricular failure and subsequent sequela. As such, restoration of sinus rhythm would be prudent.

5.1 Medical management

5.1.1 Atrial arrhythmias

Beta blockers are standard first-line therapy for rate control in patients with heart failure. Rate control with beta blockers is usually sufficient for the management of atrial arrhythmias. Digoxin may be a useful adjunct to beta blocker therapy by slowing ventricular response to the atrial arrhythmia. Calcium channel blockers are not typically used in the setting of significant systolic dysfunction.

When rate control is insufficient, then restoration and maintenance of sinus rhythm may be required. Amiodarone and dofetilide are commonly utilized for conversion to sinus rhythm in adult patients. Amiodarone is the most commonly utilized antiarrhythmic as single-agent therapy in pediatric patients with VAD [33]. Refractory cases may require amiodarone in conjunction with beta blockers, certain sodium channel blockers, or digoxin.

5.1.2 Ventricular arrhythmias

Due to the underlying condition, most patients who have received a VAD likely have an indication for beta-blockade. However, it is unclear in the pediatric population if beta-blockade is adequate for prevention of ventricular arrhythmias. Adult studies are divergent with some studies demonstrating an association with beta-blocker nonuse and ventricular arrhythmias and others showing no differences [27, 45]. Amiodarone has been identified as protective against ventricular arrhythmias amongst non-LVAD patients with ICDs, however it comes with risks of adverse effects [46]. One adult study showed improved arrhythmia-free survival in LVAD patients with ventricular arrhythmias who were started on amiodarone as secondary prevention [17]. However, when baseline amiodarone use was studied in the LVAD population, there was an increased mortality associated with its use [47]. More data are needed to assess efficacy of antiarrhythmics in the adult LVAD population and there is a near-absence in data in the pediatric population. Therefore, decisions will continue to need to be patient-specific taking into account arrhythmia burden, substrate, patient hemodynamics, drug–drug interactions, and type of VAD. Should an antiarrhythmic be initiated, as the first month post VAD implantation is reported as the highest risk [48], consideration could be made for discontinuation of antiarrhythmic medication over time in patients with longer-term VAD.

5.2 Catheter ablation

Catheter ablation of atrial arrhythmias in adult patients with heart failure has been proven to be feasible and effective [29, 49, 50]. Atrial fibrillation in setting of VAD therapy treated with catheter ablation has been associated with improved symptoms and cardiac function. Studies have demonstrated return to sinus rhythm, resolution of symptoms, and resolution of right heart failure with catheter ablation of atrial flutter in patients with VAD. No significant procedural complications or adverse events have been reported in this patient population, suggesting that radiofrequency catheter ablation of atrial arrhythmias in patients with VAD may be a reasonable first-line therapy. There are no similar data available in pediatric patients.

There have been no large studies investigating the role of catheter ablation in ventricular arrhythmias in pediatric patients with LVADs. There are a handful of adult case series and cohort studies documenting experience with 101 patients total [25]. These studies demonstrated relatively high procedural success (77–86%) with variable recurrence. One study demonstrated improved one year survival in the absence of arrhythmia recurrence [51]. It must be noted that there are specific considerations necessary for ablations in this patient population. They will require strict fluid management, invasive hemodynamic monitoring, and special care maneuvering in the vicinity of the cannula. Additionally, there may be effects on electroanatomic mapping and signal quality. Surgical ablation at the time of LVAD implant may be considered and is a class IIb indication in the 2017 guidelines for management of patients with ventricular arrhythmias and the prevention of sudden cardiac death [35]. Again, there are no published pediatric studies examining ventricular catheter ablations in patients with VADs.

5.3 Implantable cardioverter-defibrillator

ICD therapy has been demonstrated to improve survival in patients with heart failure as well as those with cardiomyopathy with previous cardiac arrests [35]. Therefore, most patients with VADs have already received an ICD or meet criteria for having one implanted. There are currently no randomized control trials evaluating ICD use in patients with VADs in adults or children. Studies investigating the effects of ICD therapy in patients with VAD have had mixed results. Early reports in the era of pulsatile VADs suggested an improvement in mortality rates in patients with ICDs [27, 52]. With the publication of studies evaluating adults with continuous flow VADs, three meta-analyses were published, with overlapping data, all with the finding that ICD use conferred no benefit in mortality risk [53–55]. Based on this, there is a class IIa recommendation for implantation of an ICD in patients with LVADs who have had ventricular arrhythmias in the 2017 AHA/ACC/HRS guidelines on ventricular arrhythmias [35]. There is no mention of VADs in the 2021 pediatric device consensus statement [36].

It is important to keep in mind that with the support of a VAD, ventricular arrhythmias may no longer cause hemodynamic compromise and patients may not lose consciousness, therefore a shock from a device may be felt. Adverse events in patients with ICDs and VADs are reported in up to 30% of patients and can include changes in thresholds, inappropriate shocks caused by oversensing, and increased defibrillation thresholds [56]. Most of these patients require an ICD modification. Programming changes should be considered in the patient with a VAD to minimize shocks in the awake patient. While studies have shown significant psychological effects of being shocked by a device versus no shock in adults, this has not been replicated in pediatrics, although limited data size may have affected the ability to detect this [57, 58]. Regardless, it is in everyone's best interest to minimize pain in our patients. A single center randomized study investigated whether lengthening detection zones and increasing the use of ATP differed from nominal settings [59]. This found no difference in time to first ICD shock, but there were no harmful effects in making these adjustments. Therefore, there have been recommendations to follow this strategy with a high rate for the VF cutoff zone and the maximum number of programmable intervals [25].

6. Conclusion

Pediatric heart failure is a complex clinical syndrome associated with high morbidity and mortality. While VAD therapy has emerged as an important tool in the management of severe or refractory heart failure, it is not uncommon to encounter arrhythmias in such patients, including during and after VAD therapy, due to the underlying pathology. To date, data on arrhythmias and arrhythmia management in the context of VADs in pediatric patients are lacking. While we have a baseline understanding of etiologies of arrhythmia substrates in patients with congenital heart disease and cardiomyopathy, the changes that occur with VAD implant are less well understood. Additionally, in pediatrics, there is evidence that new ventricular arrhythmias can present after VAD removal [11]. At this time, there is a scientific statement from the AHA that offers suggestions and recommendation for the adult population and can be a useful resource [25]. However, pediatric patients are unique and must be treated in a case-by-case basis. Maintaining sinus rhythm is clearly advantageous in the biventricular heart and can help avoid right heart failure [60]. However, in this era where fewer than 50% of pediatric patients are discharged with a VAD, one must ask how aggressively to treat these arrhythmias, especially when it comes to implanting an ICD [61]. With adult data suggesting no benefit to ICD implantation, there must be careful consideration before implanting one in a pediatric patient, especially if the patient will remain hospitalized. If an ICD is already in place, a multidisciplinary approach with the heart failure team, patient, and patient's family is necessary to determine what, if any, therapies should remain turned on when a VAD is implanted. Despite this, it is likely in the patient's best interest to avoid sustained arrhythmias and attempt to maintain appropriate heart rates to optimize VAD function, especially in single ventricle patients [41]. As technologies emerge and survival improves, the need for data to help direct management is greater than ever; however collaborative efforts will be absolutely necessary to gain the necessary knowledge.

Conflict of interest

The authors declare no conflict of interest.

Notes/thanks/other declarations

None.

Author details

Karine Guerrier[1*] and Ahmad Sami Chaouki[2]

1 Le Bonheur Children's Hospital, The University of Tennessee Health Science Center, Memphis, TN, USA

2 Ann and Robert H Lurie Children's Hospital of Chicago, Northwestern University, Feinberg School of Medicine, Chicago, USA

*Address all correspondence to: kguerrie@uthsc.edu

References

[1] Rossano JW, Kim JJ, Decker JA, Price JF, Zafar F, Graves DE, et al. Prevalence, morbidity, and mortality of heart failure-related hospitalizations in children in the United States: A population-based study. Journal of Cardiac Failure. 2012;**18**(6):459-470

[2] Lui GK, Fernandes S, McElhinney DB. Management of cardiovascular risk factors in adults with congenital heart disease. Journal of the American Heart Association. 2014;**3**(6):e001076

[3] Kantor PF, Redington AN. Pathophysiology and management of heart failure in repaired congenital heart disease. Heart Failure Clinics. 2010;**6**(4):497-506 ix

[4] Rossano JW, Shaddy RE. Heart failure in children: Etiology and treatment. The Journal of Pediatrics. 2014;**165**(2):228-233

[5] Burstein DS, Shamszad P, Dai D, Almond CS, Price JF, Lin KY, et al. Significant mortality, morbidity and resource utilization associated with advanced heart failure in congenital heart disease in children and young adults. American Heart Journal. 2019;**209**:9-19

[6] Kormos RL, Cowger J, Pagani FD, Teuteberg JJ, Goldstein DJ, Jacobs JP, et al. The Society of Thoracic Surgeons Intermacs database annual report: Evolving indications, outcomes, and scientific partnerships. The Journal of Heart and Lung Transplantation. 2019;**38**(2):114-126

[7] Mansfield RT, Lin KY, Zaoutis T, Mott AR, Mohamad Z, Luan X, et al. The use of Pediatric ventricular assist devices in Children's hospitals from 2000 to 2010: Morbidity, mortality, and hospital charges. Pediatric Critical Care Medicine. 2015;**16**(6):522-528

[8] Blume ED, Naftel DC, Bastardi HJ, Duncan BW, Kirklin JK, Webber SA, et al. Outcomes of children bridged to heart transplantation with ventricular assist devices: A multi-institutional study. Circulation. 2006;**113**(19):2313-2319

[9] Puri K, Anders MM, Tume SC, Cabrera AG, Heinle JS, Causey JC, et al. Characteristics and outcomes of Pediatric patients supported with ventricular assist device-a multi-institutional analysis. Pediatric Critical Care Medicine. 2019;**20**(8):744-752

[10] Pompa AG, Beerman LB, Feingold B, Zinn MD, Arora G. Arrhythmia burden in Pediatric patients with a ventricular assist device. Circulation. Heart Failure. 2022. 101161CIRCHEARTFAILURE 122009566

[11] Kyle WB, Decker J, Macicek SL, Valdes SO, Morales D, Hong B, et al. Arrhythmias in children with ventricular assist devices. Cardiology in the Young. 2015;**25**(2):255-260

[12] Adachi I, Burki S, Zafar F, Morales DL. Pediatric ventricular assist devices. Journal of Thoracic Disease. 2015;**7**(12):2194-2202

[13] Han JJ, Acker MA, Atluri P. Left ventricular assist devices. Circulation. 2018;**138**(24):2841-2851

[14] Adachi I, Guzman-Pruneda FA, Jeewa A, Fraser CD Jr, Dean MKE. A modified implantation technique of the HeartWare ventricular assist device for pediatric patients. The Journal

of Heart and Lung Transplantation. 2015;**34**(1):134-136

[15] Levine BD, Cornwell WK 3rd, Drazner MH. Factors influencing the rate of flow through continuous-flow left ventricular assist devices at rest and with exercise. JACC: Heart Failure. 2014;**2**(4):331-334

[16] Rosenthal DN, Almond CS, Jaquiss RD, Peyton CE, Auerbach SR, Morales DR, et al. Adverse events in children implanted with ventricular assist devices in the United States: Data from the Pediatric interagency registry for mechanical circulatory support (PediMACS). The Journal of Heart and Lung Transplantation. 2016;**35**(5):569-577

[17] Raasch H, Jensen BC, Chang PP, Mounsey JP, Gehi AK, Chung EH, et al. Epidemiology, management, and outcomes of sustained ventricular arrhythmias after continuous-flow left ventricular assist device implantation. American Heart Journal. 2012;**164**(3):373-378

[18] Carlisle MA, Fudim M, DeVore AD, Piccini JP. Heart failure and atrial fibrillation, like fire and fury. JACC: Heart Failure. 2019;**7**(6):447-456

[19] Sugumar H, Nanayakkara S, Prabhu S, Voskoboinik A, Kaye DM, Ling LH, et al. Pathophysiology of atrial fibrillation and heart failure: Dangerous interactions. Cardiology Clinics. 2019;**37**(2):131-138

[20] Sanders P, Morton JB, Davidson NC, Spence SJ, Vohra JK, Sparks PB, et al. Electrical remodeling of the atria in congestive heart failure: Electrophysiological and electroanatomic mapping in humans. Circulation. 2003;**108**(12):1461-1468

[21] Staerk L, Sherer JA, Ko D, Benjamin EJ, Helm RH. Atrial fibrillation: Epidemiology, pathophysiology, and clinical outcomes. Circulation Research. 2017;**120**(9):1501-1517

[22] Li D, Melnyk P, Feng J, Wang Z, Petrecca K, Shrier A, et al. Effects of experimental heart failure on atrial cellular and ionic electrophysiology. Circulation. 2000;**101**(22):2631-2638

[23] Efimova E, Fischer J, Bertagnolli L, Dinov B, Kircher S, Rolf S, et al. Predictors of ventricular arrhythmia after left ventricular assist device implantation: A large single-center observational study. Heart Rhythm. 2017;**14**(12):1812-1819

[24] Ebinger MW, Krishnan S, Schuger CD. Mechanisms of ventricular arrhythmias in heart failure. Current Heart Failure Reports. 2005;**2**(3):111-117

[25] Gopinathannair R, Cornwell WK, Dukes JW, Ellis CR, Hickey KT, Joglar JA, et al. Device therapy and arrhythmia Management in Left Ventricular Assist Device Recipients: A scientific statement from the American Heart Association. Circulation. 2019;**139**(20):e967-ee89

[26] Harding JD, Piacentino V 3rd, Rothman S, Chambers S, Jessup M, Margulies KB. Prolonged repolarization after ventricular assist device support is associated with arrhythmias in humans with congestive heart failure. Journal of Cardiac Failure. 2005;**11**(3):227-232

[27] Refaat M, Chemaly E, Lebeche D, Gwathmey JK, Hajjar RJ. Ventricular arrhythmias after left ventricular assist device implantation. Pacing and Clinical Electrophysiology. 2008;**31**(10):1246-1252

[28] Hayward CS, Salamonsen R, Keogh AM, Woodard J, Ayre P, Prichard R,

et al. Effect of alteration in pump speed on pump output and left ventricular filling with continuous-flow left ventricular assist device. ASAIO Journal. 2011;**57**(6):495-500

[29] Hottigoudar RU, Deam AG, Birks EJ, McCants KC, Slaughter MS, Gopinathannair R. Catheter ablation of atrial flutter in patients with left ventricular assist device improves symptoms of right heart failure. Congestive Heart Failure. 2013;**19**(4):165-171

[30] Hawkins RB, Mehaffey JH, Guo A, Charles EJ, Speir AM, Rich JB, et al. Postoperative atrial fibrillation is associated with increased morbidity and resource utilization after left ventricular assist device placement. The Journal of Thoracic and Cardiovascular Surgery. 2018;**156**(4):1543-9 e4

[31] Maisel WH, Stevenson LW. Atrial fibrillation in heart failure: Epidemiology, pathophysiology, and rationale for therapy. The American Journal of Cardiology. 2003;**91**(6A):2D-8D

[32] Blumer V, Ortiz Bezara M, Kittipibul V, Greene SJ, Fudim M, Hernandez GA, et al. Impact of atrial fibrillation on In-hospital mortality and thromboembolic complications after left ventricular assist device implantation. Journal of Cardiovascular Translational Research. 2021;**14**(1):120-124

[33] Silva JN, Erickson CC, Carter CD, Greene EA, Kantoch M, Collins KK, et al. Management of pediatric tachyarrhythmias on mechanical support. Circulation. Arrhythmia and Electrophysiology. 2014;**7**(4):658-663

[34] Houck CA, Chandler SF, Bogers A, Triedman JK, Walsh EP, de Groot NMS, et al. Arrhythmia mechanisms and outcomes of ablation in Pediatric patients with congenital heart disease. Circulation. Arrhythmia and Electrophysiology. 2019;**12**(11):e007663

[35] Al-Khatib SM, Stevenson WG, Ackerman MJ, Bryant WJ, Callans DJ, Curtis AB, et al. 2017 AHA/ACC/HRS guideline for Management of Patients with Ventricular Arrhythmias and the prevention of sudden cardiac death: A report of the American College of Cardiology/American Heart Association task force on clinical practice guidelines and the Heart Rhythm Society. Journal of the American College of Cardiology. 2018;**72**(14):e91-e220

[36] Shah MJ, Silka MJ, Silva JA, Balaji S, Beach C, Benjamin M, et al. 2021 PACES expert consensus statement on the indications and management of cardiovascular implantable electronic devices in pediatric patients. JACC: Clinical Electrophysiology. Nov 2021;**7**(11):1437-1472

[37] Magnetta DA, Reichhold A, Thrush PT, Monge M, Webster G, Joong A. Biventricular assist device support for intractable arrhythmias from histiocytoid cardiomyopathy. ASAIO Journal. Apr 15, 2022

[38] Ziv O, Dizon J, Thosani A, Naka Y, Magnano AR, Garan H. Effects of left ventricular assist device therapy on ventricular arrhythmias. Journal of the American College of Cardiology. 2005;**45**(9):1428-1434

[39] Berg DD, Vaduganathan M, Upadhyay GA, Singh JP, Mehra MR, Stewart GC. Cardiac implantable electronic devices in patients with left ventricular assist systems. Journal of the American College of Cardiology. 2018;**71**(13):1483-1493

[40] Oz MC, Rose EA, Slater J, Kuiper JJ, Catanese KA, Levin HR. Malignant

ventricular arrhythmias are well tolerated in patients receiving long-term left ventricular assist devices. Journal of the American College of Cardiology. 1994;**24**(7):1688-1691

[41] Lorts A, Conway J, Schweiger M, Adachi I, Amdani S, Auerbach SR, et al. ISHLT consensus statement for the selection and management of pediatric and congenital heart disease patients on ventricular assist devices endorsed by the American Heart Association. The Journal of Heart and Lung Transplantation. 2021;**40**(8):709-732

[42] Baldwin ACW, Gemmato CJ, Sandoval E, Cohn WE, Morgan JA, Frazier OH. Tolerance of sustained ventricular fibrillation during continuous-flow left ventricular assist device support. Texas Heart Institute Journal. 2017;**44**(5):357-360

[43] Jakstaite AM, Luedike P, Wakili R, Kochhauser S, Ruhparwar A, Rassaf T, et al. Case report: incessant ventricular fibrillation in a conscious left ventricular assist device patient. European Heart Journal - Case Reports. 2021;**5**(9):ytab337

[44] Smith ME, Moak JH. Asymptomatic ventricular fibrillation in continuous flow left-ventricular assist device. The American Journal of Emergency Medicine. 2021;**49**:130-132

[45] Andersen M, Videbaek R, Boesgaard S, Sander K, Hansen PB, Gustafsson F. Incidence of ventricular arrhythmias in patients on long-term support with a continuous-flow assist device (HeartMate II). The Journal of Heart and Lung Transplantation. 2009;**28**(7):733-735

[46] Santangeli P, Muser D, Maeda S, Filtz A, Zado ES, Frankel DS, et al. Comparative effectiveness of antiarrhythmic drugs and catheter ablation for the prevention of recurrent ventricular tachycardia in patients with implantable cardioverter-defibrillators: A systematic review and meta-analysis of randomized controlled trials. Heart Rhythm. 2016;**13**(7):1552-1559

[47] Gopinathannair R, Roukoz H, Bhan A, Ravichandran A, Ahmed MM, Familtsev D, et al. Cardiac resynchronization therapy and clinical outcomes in continuous flow left ventricular assist device recipients. Journal of the American Heart Association. Jun 15, 2018;**7**(12):1-10

[48] Healy C, Viles-Gonzalez JF, Sacher F, Coffey JO, d'Avila A. Management of Ventricular Arrhythmias in patients with mechanical ventricular support devices. Current Cardiology Reports. 2015;**17**(8):59

[49] Chung YJ, Choi JO, Park KM. Catheter ablation for atrial fibrillation in left ventricular assist device: A case report. Medicine (Baltimore). 2021;**100**(25):e26308

[50] Maury P, Delmas C, Trouillet C, Slaughter MS, Lairez O, Galinier M, et al. First experience of percutaneous radio-frequency ablation for atrial flutter and atrial fibrillation in a patient with HeartMate II left ventricular assist device. Journal of Interventional Cardiac Electrophysiology. 2010;**29**(1):63-67

[51] Moss JD, Flatley EE, Beaser AD, Shin JH, Nayak HM, Upadhyay GA, et al. Characterization of ventricular tachycardia after left ventricular assist device implantation as destination therapy: A single-Center ablation experience. JACC: Clinical Electrophysiology. 2017;**3**(12):1412-1424

[52] Cantillon DJ, Tarakji KG, Kumbhani DJ, Smedira NG, Starling RC, Wilkoff BL. Improved survival among

ventricular assist device recipients with a concomitant implantable cardioverter-defibrillator. Heart Rhythm. 2010;**7**(4):466-471

[53] Agrawal S, Garg L, Nanda S, Sharma A, Bhatia N, Manda Y, et al. The role of implantable cardioverter-defibrillators in patients with continuous flow left ventricular assist devices - a meta-analysis. International Journal of Cardiology. 2016;**222**:379-384

[54] Elkaryoni A, Badarin FA, Khan MS, Ellakany K, Potturi N, Poonia J, et al. Implantable cardioverter-defibrillators and survival in advanced heart failure patients with continuous-flow left ventricular assist devices: A systematic review and meta-analysis. Europace. 2019;**21**(9):1353-1359

[55] Vakil K, Kazmirczak F, Sathnur N, Adabag S, Cantillon DJ, Kiehl EL, et al. Implantable cardioverter-defibrillator use in patients with left ventricular assist devices: A systematic review and Meta-analysis. JACC: Heart Failure. 2016;**4**(10):772-779

[56] Thomas IC, Cork DP, Levy A, Nayak H, Beshai JF, Burke MC, et al. ICD lead parameters, performance, and adverse events following continuous-flow LVAD implantation. Pacing and Clinical Electrophysiology. 2014;**37**(4):464-472

[57] Gopinathannair R, Lerew DR, Cross NJ, Sears SF, Brown S, Olshansky B. Longitudinal changes in quality of life following ICD implant and the impact of age, gender, and ICD shocks: Observations from the INTRINSIC RV trial. Journal of Interventional Cardiac Electrophysiology. 2017;**48**(3):291-298

[58] Sears SF, Hazelton AG, St Amant J, Matchett M, Kovacs A, Vazquez LD, et al. Quality of life in pediatric patients with implantable cardioverter defibrillators. The American Journal of Cardiology. 2011;**107**(7):1023-1027

[59] Richardson TD, Hale L, Arteaga C, Xu M, Keebler M, Schlendorf K, et al. Prospective randomized evaluation of implantable cardioverter-defibrillator programming in patients with a left ventricular assist device. Journal of the American Heart Association. Feb 23, 2018;**7**(5):1-8

[60] Law SP, Morales DLS, Si MS, Friedland-Little JM, Joong A, Bearl DW, et al. Right heart failure considerations in pediatric ventricular assist devices. Pediatric Transplantation. 2021;**25**(3):e13990

[61] Rossano JW, VanderPluym CJ, Peng DM, Hollander SA, Maeda K, Adachi I, et al. Fifth annual Pediatric interagency registry for mechanical circulatory support (Pedimacs) report. The Annals of Thoracic Surgery. 2021;**112**(6):1763-1774

Chapter 4

Implantable Cardioverter-Defibrillator Use in Patients with Left Ventricular Assist Devices

David Garcia-Molinero and Rocio Toro

Abstract

This chapter is developed with the intention of discussing the use of implantable defibrillator cardioverters (ICDs) in patients with left ventricular assist devices (LVADs). LVADs have become the standard treatment for patients with advanced heart failure who require prolonged mechanical circulatory support as a bridge to transplantation or as destination therapy. Patients with advanced heart failure have a major risk of sudden death due to ventricular dysrhythmias (VD) so an ICD could be indicated, but it remains unclear within the LVAD population due to several factors including sustained VD good tolerance and inappropriate therapies (due to supraventricular tachycardias or electromechanical interferences) as well as the risk of infections with complex antibiotic therapy or device replacements. Previous VD before LVAD placement, concomitant atrial fibrillation, type of LVAD device, and chronic ischemic heart disease can predict future episodes of VD. The evidence that supports ICD use in patients with LVAD is very limited, and current guidelines are based primarily on the consensus of experts and observational studies. Nowadays, an ICD implant is only recommended for LVAD patients who develop postoperative VD associated with hemodynamic collapse, and it should be programmed in a very conservative mode (higher rate and larger intervals to detection) to avoid undesirable electric shocks.

Keywords: implanted cardioverter defibrillator, ventricular assist device, ventricular arrhythmia, advanced heart failure, sudden death

1. Introduction

Left ventricular assist devices (LVADs) have become the standard treatment for patients with advanced heart failure who require prolonged mechanical circulatory support as a bridge to transplantation or as destination therapy [1–5]. The first generation of LVAD consisted of pulsatile pumps that were successful in unloading the heart, but they were limited by size and poor long-term durability. The second and third generations use continuous flow (i.e., Heartware or Heartmate II devices). Heartmate III is nowadays the only third-generation device available to implant due to its magnetic levitation rotor related to lower rates of thrombus and hemolysis. One-year survival rates are approximately 80% and 70% at 2 years [4].

Patients with advanced HF have a major risk of sudden death due to ventricular dysrhythmias (VD). Therefore, an implantable cardioverter defibrillator (ICD) could be indicated. Primary prevention needs the device prescription before a fatal episode and is indicated if severe LVEF dysfunction (less than 35%) is diagnosed using any cardiac imaging tool such as transthoracic echocardiography or cardiac magnetic resonance, 40 days after myocardial infarction, despite full-medical protocol, the patient is not stable and if the estimation of the patient survival is more than 1 year. On the other hand, the secondary is indicated after ventricular arrhythmia [3, 6–9].

Patients in stage D often die of pump failure rather than sudden death, so ICD therapies have not been recommended in this population. Cardiac output impairment is less common [10] in LVAD subjects, and VD is better tolerated [3] than in the non-LVAD population. Moreover, inappropriate therapies and complex infections may increase the risk of ICD therapy. Therefore, ICD therapies remain controversial in the LVAD population, and further research is needed.

2. Epidemiology of ventricular arrhythmia and cardiac sudden death

The highest rates of VD occur in the first 30 days after LVAD placement; however, late ventricular dysrhythmias have also been described. VD incidence ranges from 22% to 59% after LVAD implant [10–12] and 35% of post-LVAD recipients within 30 days [13, 14].

Several factors can predict VD events after LVAD implantation, i.e., previous ventricular dysrhythmias before LVAD implant (hazard ratio 3.28) [15], previous history of atrial fibrillation [14–16], the type of LVAD implanted, or the presence concomitant chronic ischemic heart disease [17]. In total, 42.4% of patients with a history of VD pre-LVAD experienced VD events post-LVAD in comparison with 16.7% without previous VD [12]. Ischemic heart disease was the major cause of cardiomyopathy in 71% of patients in the VD group and 45% of patients in the group without VD where dilated cardiomyopathy was more frequent (no difference was made between inheriting cardiomyopathy, enolic, cardiotoxicity, or idiopathic cause). Chronic ischemic heart disease could trigger VD due to persistent subendocardial ischemia, arrhythmogenic substrate associated with myocyte remodeling, and fibrosis [17].

VD often leads to sudden cardiac death in the non-LVAD population. However, long-term survival has been reported in those patients with LVADs despite VD [11]. Interestingly, neither the presence of VD nor ICD therapies (appropriate in 19.1% or inappropriate in 3.1%) were associated with higher mortality rates after 10 months of follow-up [15].

Controversially, other studies have described higher mortality in patients with VD events. Bedi et al. showed an absolute 15% or higher risk of death in the first week after LVAD implantation [17]. Brenyo et al. describe an increase in mortality of up to 10 times higher in patients with LVADs if there is concomitant VD, although 1 year of mean follow-up makes it difficult to correlate VD as a cause of death or as a progression marker of disease [18].

3. Mechanisms and management of ventricular dysrhythmias

The mechanisms of VD in LVAD include:

1. The perioperative adrenergic stimulation and adrenergic agonists may promote early VD [14] because of myocardial or systemic inflammation after LVAD implant, which can elevate catecholamine blood level and promote changes in electrical properties making LV more sensitive to VD. Indeed, isoproterenol, norepinephrine, and dobutamine are treatments often used to avoid RV failure during the perioperative time; however, they can also help to achieve an electrical imbalance and generate a VD substrate.

2. The cardiomyopathy severity, above all, chronic ischemic disease is related to the presence of intrinsic scars that perpetuate reentrant circuits and VD [14].

3. The apical insertion site of cannula inflow has been correlated to the morphological origin of ventricular tachycardia [14]. Although 75% of ventricular tachycardia mapped during electrophysiological studies correlated to an intrinsic scar [19] unrelated to the device.

4. The suction events, an excessive left ventricular discharge due to a mismatch between LVEF filling and LVAD output. When LVEF is excessively unloaded, it can collapse and lead to VD event, monomorphic or polymorphic. But also, an inadequate left ventricular discharge can promote VD [14].

5. The type of LVAD can predict the risk of VD. There was a significant twofold increase in risk for LVAD versus biventricular-VAD [20]. Continuous flow (CF) pumps compared with pulsatile pumps could increase the incidence of VD [21], but it could be related to suction events, more frequent in CF-LVAD due to continuous ventricular unloading.

6. Acute mechanical unloading of the LVEF during recent postoperative time can change electrophysiological properties such as an increase in QT segment within 1 week after LVAD and a decrease after 1 week of mechanical support. A longer QT segment after LVAD placement has been associated with a threefold higher risk for postoperative VD [14].

In a multivariate analysis, VD after LVAD placement in the recent perioperative time was associated with a higher risk of all-cause mortality compared with the population without VD (hazard ratio 7.28). This report suggests that aggressive treatment must be considered [16].

Three main treatment options exist, including adjusting LVAD settings, medical treatment, and VT ablation.

Suction events are a common trigger for ventricular arrhythmias in patients with LVAD; therefore, reduction in LVAD speed or an increase in intravascular volume could solve VD. Once preload and unload are assessed, the next line of treatment should be medical therapy.

Limited literature suggests any potential benefit from the use of β-blockers, amiodarone, sotalol (take care of changes in QT), and sodium channel blockers (lidocaine/mexiletine); but these potential treatments need further studying [14]. A correct repositioning of potassium and magnesium ions is also required.

Radiofrequency ablation therapy has been described as an alternative option in some reports with low complication rates when VD persists, and there is a hemodynamic compromise or a worsening of RV function [13].

If there is prior history of ventricular dysrhythmias in LVAD candidates, surgical ablation at the time of LVAD placement should be considered, as it offers direct visualization of the myocardium and epicardial ablation without defects of epicardial mapping and ablation *via* subxiphoid pericardial access. Endocardial electroanatomic mapping before the LVAD implantation procedure may let localize VD circuits and guide surgical planning. Once LVAD has been placed, options for ablation of VD are more limited due to pericardial adhesions from the device, and LVAD inflow cannula limits endocardial access to the LV apex.

If catheter ablation is planned, several anatomic and physiologic challenges must be considered. Retrograde access can be limited by insufficient native flow to open the aortic valve, so a transseptal approach to the left ventricle (through the left atrium) is the preferred option. The LVAD often causes magnetic interference that may affect mapping systems.

Nonetheless, a recent systematic review of 18 studies showed that catheter ablation was associated with a decrease in rates of ICD therapies (57 vs. 24%), but VD recurred in 44% at a mean follow-up of 264 days [22].

4. Ventricular arrhythmia tolerance and Fontan-type circulation

LVAD population has a better tolerance for sustained VD, including ventricular fibrillation (VF) than the non-LVAD population, most likely due to the "Fontan-type circulation" phenomena. This population has the same ability to withstand insults as patients with congenital heart diseases and Fontan-type circulation [3] described by Fontan and Baudet in 1971 to palliate tricuspid atresia relying on central venous circulation enabling blood to be directed toward the RV in the absence of pulmonary hypertension.

In patients with LVAD, the right ventricle behaves as a passive corridor driving blood from right to left if adequate preload condition is met. High pulmonary pressure or low central venous pressure is associated with more difficulties to remain stable once VD appears [23, 24].

Sims et al. [25] described how a continuous flow-LVAD could avoid collapse in a patient with sustained ventricular fibrillation over 12 hours when an implantable defibrillator was not able to terminate arrhythmia and external defibrillation was required, due to a correct preload to the LV and normal or low pulmonary resistances. The same findings were described by Busch et al. and Smith et al. [26, 27].

5. Evidence for implantable cardioverter defibrillator device

The evidence that supports ICD indication in patients with LVAD is very limited, and current guidelines are based primarily on the consensus of experts and observational studies [13].

A meta-analysis by Vakil et al. showed that ICD therapy was associated with an absolute risk reduction of 16% and a relative risk reduction of 39% in all-cause mortality at a 7-month follow-up. The number of patients who needed to treat to avoid an outcome was six subjects [11]. Nevertheless, there is not any statistical significance in the continuous-flow LVAD subgroup (34% of the total population). The ICD cohort showed a mortality up to 14% vs. 25% in the non-ICD group (and an absolute risk reduction of 11% and a 24% relative risk (p = 0.17). The lack of significant results was due to the small sample size due to the better long-term results and hemodynamic stability with new continuous-flow assistance [13] with less dependence on native cardiac activity than pulsatile pumps [28].

Rorris et al. did not find any difference in all-cause mortality events, cardiovascular mortality, or right heart failure between LVAD patients with and without an ICD. Although, the study finds important differences in baseline patient characteristics between European and United States populations [29].

A subanalysis of the INTERMACS Registry that included of 2209 patients with an ICD and 2209 patients without one concluded that the presence of ICD was not related to reduced mortality, among patients with a continuous-flow LVAD. The presence of an ICD was associated with increased mortality risk and unexpected death during device support because of the result of propensity score matching, which resulted in an ICD group that had decreased prevalence of certain VD risk factors (as beta-blocker or amiodarone use, prior to VD, or chronic HF) [28].

Kutyfa et al. demonstrated that neither implant ICD before nor after LVAD reached significant survival benefit in a 191-patient study after 23 months of follow-up [30].

Younes et al. designed a 1444 patients study included in a waitlist HF bridged to transplant with LVAD. These authors suggested that the presence of ICD was not associated with lower mortality, cardiovascular or global mortality, or delisting although arrhythmic death was more common in the non-ICD group compared with ICD [12, 31].

A 94-patient study about the use of ICD after continuous-flow LVAD implant showed that only patients with VD before LVAD placement had any benefit [19]. Therefore, it is reasonable to not implant ICD in LVAD patients without previous VD [20].

Alvarez et al. [3] studied 487 patients, mostly with ICDS, 79.6%. The presence of ICD before LVAD was not related to a significant benefit in terms of mortality. However, ICD patients before LVAD presented complications such as episodes of shocks (31%), ventricular lead dysfunction (4.6%), and 2% of infections associated with ICD [3, 32].

The high rates of inappropriate shocks and infection events may decrease the benefits of the ICD indication [5]. Indeed, ICD shocks are associated with worse long-term outcomes and poorer quality of life and can negatively affect mental status [33]. Patients experience inappropriate shocks due to supraventricular tachycardias or electromagnetic interference; for that reason; benefit of appropriate shocks for prolonged but hemodynamically critical VD remains unclear [12].

Infection is a frequent complication in the LVAD population (i.e., driveline infection or device-related sepsis) that can occur in up to 20% of patients. Malnutrition and high comorbidity including diabetes, surgical technique, and quality of percutaneous lead care are important risk factors for infection. Aggressive management often is needed including long-term antibiotics, device exchange, or even urgent transplants [4]. Therefore, infection treatment could be more complex in the presence of both devices (LVAD and ICD).

Riaz et al. described a cohort of 215 ICD-LVAD patients and six (2.8%) developed ICD infections. Three patients had pocket infections related to device generator exchange, and three patients had ICD lead-related endocarditis due to prior LVAD-related infections. In all cases, ICD was removed along with antibiotics. Three patients with a history of previous LVAD infections received longer antimicrobial therapy, and one patient had their LVAD exchanged [32].

Finally, at the last 2019 EACTS Expert Consensus on long-term mechanical circulatory support [34] indications are: (i) patients with LVAD who develop postoperative ventricular dysrhythmias associated with hemodynamic collapse, ICD implantation is

2019 EACTS Expert Consensus on long-term mechanical circulatory support		
In patients with long-term mechanical circulatory support who develop postoperative ventricular arrhythmia with hemodynamic compromise, ICD implantation is recommended.	I	C
To prevent adverse sequelae of right ventricular dysfunction, a continuation of ICD therapy should be considered.	IIa	C
Prophylactic ICD implantation in patients without arrhythmias at the time of long-term mechanical circulatory support implantation is not recommended.	III	C
2022 ESC Guidelines for the management of patients with ventricular arrhythmias and the prevention of sudden cardiac death		
ICD implantation should be considered in LVAD recipients with symptomatic sustained VAs.	IIa	B

Table 1.
Summary of current guidelines about the use of implantable cardioverter defibrillator devices in the LVAD population.

recommended (IC); (ii) patients who have an ICD implanted before LVAD, it should be kept activated for prevention of adverse effects due to right ventricular dysfunction, but its programming should be very conservative (IIaC); (iii) primary prevention is not recommended in patients without VD before LVAD (IIIC).

On the other hand, the 2022 ESC Guidelines for the management of patients with ventricular dysrhythmias and the prevention of sudden cardiac death [35] recommends: ICD implantation should be considered in LVAD recipients with symptomatic sustained VD (IIaB) **Table 1**.

6. How to program implantable cardioverter defibrillator devices

Current guidelines recommend conservative programming for ICD [34–37] based on good tolerance of VD and high rates of inappropriate shocks due to atrial tachycardia (AT), including atrial fibrillation (high rates in HF patients).

Richardson et al. [10] carry out an 83-patient randomized study (well-balanced between ischemic and non-ischemic cardiomyopathy) divided into a first standard programming arm according to the treating physician (**Table 2**) and a second ultra-conservative ICD mode (**Table 3**).

As it is known, detection to rate and intervals to detection are important parameters to program an ICD to achieve the highest benefit and to avoid inappropriate shocks. The first one is related to the range of heart rate where ICD acts, and intervals are the numbers of cycles or time to detect before applying therapies. As **Table 1** shows, different therapy zones can be chosen, e.g., VT zone or VT1, VT2/VF zone, and VF zone based on these parameters to reach the optimal status for the patient. These zones must be correlated to patient profile, for instance, ischemic cardiomyopathy vs. myocardiopathy and primary vs. secondary prevention.

As indicated in **Table 3**, the ultra-conservative mode uses larger intervals of detection in the VF and VT zones and numerous anti-tachycardia pacing programming (ATP) therapies than the standard mode.

No difference related to time to the first ICD shock or the total number of shocks was found between the two groups. No statistical difference was observed in mortality terms, arrhythmic events, or heart failure hospitalization events. Inappropriate

VF zone active	38 patients (100%)
Detection to rate	214 bpm (200–228)
Intervals to detection	16 (12–24)
VT zone active	26 patients (68%)
Detection rate	176 (167–181)
Intervals to detection	19 (16–27)
FV/VT-2 zone active	9 patients (24%)
Detection to rate	187 (182–188)
Intervals to detection	24 (18–30)

VF: ventricular fibrillation, VT: ventricular tachycardia, bpm: beats per minute.

Table 2.
Adapted from Richardson et al. shows the programming values of ICD in the standard mode.

Manufacturer	VT zone detection	VI zone therapy	VF zone detection	VF zone therapy
Medtronic Inc.	Rate: 180 bpm 100 intervals (33 s) to detection	ATP × 5; 25 J × 2	Rate: 222 bpm 120/160 intervals to detection (32,4s)	25 J, 35 J × 5
Boston Scientific Inc.	Rate 180 bpm 30 s to detection	ATP × 8, 21 J, 41 J × 6	Rate: 220 bpm 15 s to detection	29 J, 41 J × 7
St. Jude Medical	Rate 180 bpm 100 intervals (33 s) to detection	ATP × 3, 36 J, 40 J × 2	Rate: 240 bpm 100 intervals to detection (25 s)	36 J, 40 J × 5

ATP: anti-tachycardia pacing, J: Joules.

Table 3.
Adapted from Richardson et al. shows the programming values of the ICD in the ultraconservative mode.

shocks resulted in 6% of the total population, although no significant differences between both groups were found [10].

However, the MADIT-RIT study showed fewer inappropriate shocks and lower all-cause mortality in those patients scheduled for ICD therapies greater than 200 bpm [38]. This study compared conventional programming versus another more conservative population with prior AT and patients without prior AT and described a statistical reduction of inappropriate shocks with conservative programming able.

Moreover, a randomized ADVANCE III trial (1902 patients) also demonstrated that larger detection intervals (30 of 40 intervals) decreased therapies delivered and inappropriate shocks without difference in mortality or arrhythmic syncope events compared with standard detection (18 of 24 intervals) in not LVAD carriers [39].

7. Resynchronization therapy on ventricular dysrhythmias after LVAD devices

Cardiac resynchronization therapy (CRT) is recommended for symptomatic patients with HF and a QRS duration ≥150 ms and left branch bundle block QRS morphology with LVEF ≤35% despite optical treatment can improve ventricular remodel to improve symptoms and reduce morbidity and mortality [1]. Nevertheless, its potential benefit or antiarrhythmic effect in LVAD patients remains unclear.

A prospective single-center study indicates a lower incidence of implantable cardioverter defibrillator device (ICD) therapies in the LVAD population if CRT mode was activated [40]. Richardson et al. [10] and Gopinathannair et al. [41] failed to find any differences in terms of mortality and hospitalization, but the first one corroborates the lower ICD discharges in the CRT-activated group, which could benefit from the antiarrhythmic effect of CRT.

The lack of additive effect from CRT in the LVAD population could be explained for several reasons including (i) LV unloading by LVAD surpasses the electrical correction by CRT; (ii) CRT population had a more advanced myocardiopathy to begin limiting any additive effect; (iii) CRT could improve clinical outcomes in younger patients with nonischemic dilated cardiomyopathy who receive LVAD as a bridge to recovery, but this population was not included. Muratsu et al. describe a case report of a 15-year-old male with acute decompensated heart failure and LVAD implantation as a bridge to recovery. Despite optimal treatment, a CRT was required to improve cardiac function and finally perform LVAD removal [41, 42].

More randomized studies are necessary to better know the mechanism and the benefit of maintaining CRT turned on in the LVAD population despite its use being associated with higher generator replacement rates [3].

8. Electromagnetic interactions between implantable cardioverter defibrillator and left ventricular assist devices

Both Heartware and HeartMate III (HM3) ventricular assist devices developed an electromagnetic interference (EMI) that can it make impossible to interrogate ICD with external programmers.

EMI can be explained by a pulse-width modulator (PWM), which can emit frequencies of 8 kHz, the same frequency that Abbot and Biotronik ICD/CRT programmers emit to start reading ICD. Distance between the LVAD and the ICD programmer and the speed of the LVAD rotor can also interfere [43]. HM3 manufacturing website itself provides information on possible incompatibilities (**Table 4**) [44].

Manufacturer	Family / model
Biotronik	Acticor/ Rivacor
Biotronik	Ilivia Neo/Intica Neo
Biotronik	Ilivia/Intica/Inlexa
Biotronik	Itrevia/Iperia/Inventra
Biotronik	Iforia/Ilesto/Idova
Biotronik	Lumax
ELA Medical (Sorin)	Paradyme CRT
Medtronic	Cardia CRT
Boston Scientific	ORIGEN CRT

Table 4.
Adapted from Cardiovascular Abbott. The difficulty or inability to communicate with the external programmer has been reported for or may occur with the following manufacturer families by using HM3.

Schnegg et al. [43] analyzed *in vitro* the programming of 24 explanted ICDs from several manufacturers in the presence of a running LVAD (Heartware and HM3 LVAD). Heartware LVAD interaction was only observed in the case of Biotronik and Microport devices if the distance was shorter than 6 cm, while HM3 LVAD only Medtronic ICD devices showed no interaction (needing up to 18 cm with some Biotronik devices).

Three different strategies were tested to improve connectivity between the ICD programmer and ICD: (1) Pseudo-faraday cage to achieve electromagnetic isolation of the ICD. The isolation of the ICD device with a metal pan (pseudo-faraday cage) was not effective in those devices that had previously failed (Boston and Biotronik devices); (2) LVAD parameters modification (above all speed of rotor). Once the speed of HM3 was significantly changed (−2000 rpm, +1000 rpm), communication improved up to 45% of total devices, but 55% remained unchanged; and (3) to increase the distance between LVAD and ICD by separating the arm from the thorax. This latter option, separating the arm from the thorax by bringing the hand over the head to increase the distance between ICD and LVAD, was the most effective measure. An increase of 3 cm was achieved. This posture should be maintained for the first 2–10 seconds, and then the arm can be repositioned. Alternatively, the ICD may be removed to the contralateral side as the last solution, but given the doubtful benefit of therapies in LVAD patients, it is not usually carried out [43].

A retrospective single-center study carried out by Yalcin et al. confirmed that the EMI from the Heartmate II LVAD was only present in patients with a St Jude/Abbott device (6 of the 23 St Jude/Abbott devices. In HM3 patients, EMI was mainly present in patients with Biotronik devices: four out of the 18 and only one patient with a Medtronic device. While initial interrogation of these devices was not successful, none of the 11 cases experienced pacing inhibition or inappropriate shocks [45].

Although, two studies reported a decrease in ventricular sensing with a smaller R-wave amplitude, an impedance decrease, and a capture threshold increase after LVAD placement that could lead to failure of ventricular dysrhythmias sensing, capturing failure, and inappropriate pacing [46–48]. It should be noted that the proximity of the ICD to the LVAD controller did not affect the programming values of the ICD or the shock therapies [43, 46, 49].

Black-Maier et al. describe several major findings in a systematic review of subcutaneous-ICD after LVAD implantation: ventricular sensing amplitudes reduction, EMI appears in primary and secondary vectors that lead to inappropriate shocks (above all in the postoperative period) but rarely in alternate vector, and parameters improved spontaneously during follow-up without need for device revision or extraction [50]. However, Lopez Gil et al. [51] describe a case of a 24-year-old man implanted with an S-ICD because of idiopathy dilated cardiomyopathy and self-limiting sustained VT. After the placement of an HM3, the S-ICD became useless because of inadequate sensing due to EMI and reduced QRS voltage.

9. Conclusion

There is not enough evidence to recommend the use of ICD in patients with LVAD because cardiac output impairment is less common, and VD is better tolerated than in the non-LVAD population.

The presence of VD and ischemic cardiomyopathy is a major risk for suffering VD events after an LVAD implant. VD usually occurs in the early period, the first month after placement, and they usually have good tolerance due to Fontan-like circulation physiology. Although, up to 45% of patients experience symptoms, and 24% required cardioversion or defibrillation. But only up to 4% suffer syncope or 2% required support with RVAD.

Current guidelines are based on expert consensus and observational studies recommend ICD in the LVAD population if concomitant postoperative ventricular dysrhythmias associated with hemodynamic collapse are present, and its programming should be very conservative to avoid inappropriate shocks due to AT.

Until ICD therapies have been more thoroughly investigated and have shown significant evidence to benefit LVAD patients, there will be resistance to deactivating ICD, particularly in patient's bridge to transplant.

Conflict of interest

The authors have no conflicts of interest to declare.

Author details

David Garcia-Molinero[1*] and Rocio Toro[2]

1 Puerta del Mar University Hospital, Cadiz, Spain

2 Cadiz University, Spain

*Address all correspondence to: dgmoliner@gmail.com

References

[1] Mcdonagh TA, Metra M, Adamo M, Gardner RS, Baumbach A, et al. 2021 ESC Guidelines for the diagnosis and treatment of acute and chronic heart failure: Developed by the Task Force for the diagnosis and treatment of acute and chronic heart failure of the European Society of Cardiology (ESC) With the special contribution of the Heart Failure Association (HFA) of the ESC. European Heart Journal. 2021;**42**(36):3599-3726

[2] Heidenreich PA, Bozkurt B, Aguilar D, Allen LA, Byun JJ, Colvin MM, et al. AHA/ACC/HFSA Guideline for the Management of Heart Failure: A Report of the American College of Cardiology/American Heart Association Joint Committee on Clinical Practice Guidelines. Circulation. 2022;**145**:e895-e1032

[3] Alvarez PA, Sperry BW, Pérez AL, Yaranov DM, Randhawa V, Luthman J, et al. Implantable cardioverter defibrillators in patients with continuous flow left ventricular assist devices: Utilization patterns, related procedures, and complications. Journal of the American Heart Association. 2019;**8**(14):e011813

[4] Joyce E, Starling RC. HFrEF Other Treatment: Ventricular Assist Devices. In: Camm AJ, et al, editors. The ESC Textbook of Cardiovascular Medicine, 3 edn, The European Society of Cardiology Series, Online edn. Oxford: ESC Publications; 1 Jul 2018. DOI: 10.1093/med/9780198784906.003.0432

[5] Kadakia S, Moore R, Ambur V, Toyoda Y. Current status of the implantable LVAD. General Thoracic and Cardiovascular Surgery. 2016;**64**(9):501-508. DOI: 10.1007/s11748-016-0671-y

[6] Moss AJ, Zareba W, Hall WJ, Klein H, Wilber DJ, Cannom DS, et al. Prophylactic implantation of a defibrillator in patients with myocardial infarction and reduced ejection fraction. New England Journal of Medicine. 2002;**346**(12):877-883

[7] Antiarrhythmics versus Implantable Defibrillators (AVID) Investigators. A comparison of antiarrhythmic-drug therapy with implantable defibrillators in patients resuscitated from near-fatal ventricular dysrhythmias. New England Journal of Medicine. 1997;**337**(22):1576-1583

[8] Russo AM, Stainback RF, Bailey SR, Epstein AE, Heidenreich PA, Jessup M, et al. ACCF/HRS/AHA/ASE/HFSA/SCAI/SCCT/SCMR 2013 appropriate use criteria for implantable cardioverter-defibrillators and cardiac resynchronization therapy: A report of the American College of Cardiology Foundation appropriate use criteria task force, Heart Rhythm Society, American HeartAssociation, American Society of Echocardiography, Heart Failure Society of America, Society for Cardiovascular Angiography and Interventions, Society of CardiovascularComputed Tomography, and Society for Cardiovascular Magnetic Resonance. Heart Rhythm. 2013;**10**:e11-e58

[9] Bardy GH, Lee KL, Mark DB, et al. Amiodarone or an implantable cardioverter defibrillator for congestive heart failure. New England Journal of Medicine. 2005;**352**:225-237

[10] Richardson TD, Hale L, Arteaga C, Xu M, Keebler M, Schlendorf K, et al. Prospective randomized evaluation of implantable cardioverter-defibrillator programming in patients with a left

ventricular assist device. Journal of the American Heart Association. 2005;**7**(5):e007748

[11] Vakil K, Kazmirczak F, Sathnur N, Adabag S, Cantillon DJ, Kiehl EL, et al. Implantable cardioverter-defibrillator use in patients with left ventricular assist devices. JACC: Heart Failure. 2016;**4**(10):772-779

[12] Agrawal S, Garg L, Nanda S, Sharma A, Bhatia N, Manda Y, et al. The role of implantable cardioverter-defibrillators in patients with continuous-flow left ventricular assist devices – a meta-analysis. International Journal of Cardiology. 2016;**222**:379-384. DOI: 10.1016/j.ijcard.2016.07.257

[13] Cantillon DJ, Tarakji KG, Kumbhani DJ, Smedira NG, Starling RC, Wilkoff BL. Improved survival among ventricular assist device recipients with a concomitant implantable cardioverter-defibrillator. Heart Rhythm. 2010;**7**(4):466-471. DOI: 10.1016/j.hrthm.2009.12.022

[14] Nakahara S, Chien C, Gelow J, Dalouk K, Henrikson CA, Mudd J, et al. Ventricular dysrhythmias after left ventricular assist device. Circulation Arrhythm Electrophysiology. 2013;**6**(3):648-654. DOI: 10.1161/CIRCEP.113.000113

[15] Kumar A, Tandon V, O'Sullivan DM, Cronin E, Gluck J, Kluger J. ICD shocks in LVAD patients are not associated with increased subsequent mortality risk. Journal of Interventional Cardio Electrophysiology. 2019;**56**(3):341-348. DOI: 10.1007/s10840-019-00619-7

[16] Yoruk A, Sherazi S, Massey HT, Kutyifa V, McNitt S, Hallinan W, et al. Predictors and clinical relevance of ventricular tachyarrhythmias in ambulatory patients with a continuous flow left ventricular assist device. Heart Rhythm. 2016;**13**:1052-1105. DOI: 10.1016/j.hrthm.2016.01.033

[17] Bedi M, Kormos R, Winowich S, McNamara DM, Mathier MA, Murali S. Ventricular dysrhythmias during left ventricular assist device support. The American Journal of Cardiology. 2007;**99**:1151-1153. DOI: 10.1016/j.amjcard.2006.11.051

[18] Brenyo A, Rao M, Koneru S, et al. Risk of mortality for ventricular arrhythmia in ambulatory LVAD patients. Journal of Cardiovascular Electrophysiology. 2012;**23**:515-520. DOI: 10.1111/j.1540-8167.2011.02223.x

[19] Garan AR, Yuzefpolskaya M, Colombo PC, et al. Ventricular dysrhythmias and implantable cardioverter-defibrillator therapy in patients with continuous-flow left ventricular assist devices: The need for primary prevention? Journal of the American College of Cardiology. 2013;**61**:2542-2550. DOI: 10.1016/j.jacc.2013.04.020

[20] Genovese EA, Dew MA, Teuteberg JJ, Simon MA, Kay J, Siegenthaler MP, et al. Incidence and patterns of adverse event onset during the first 60 days after ventricular assist device implantation. The Annals of Thoracic Surgery. 2009;**88**:1162-1170. DOI: 10.1016/j.athoracsur.2009.06.028

[21] Cao X, Haft J, Dyke DB, Wright S, Pagani FD, Aaronson KD. Increased incidence of ventricular tachycardia following left ventricular assist device implantation with continuous flow rotary pumps. Journal of Cardiac Failure. 2006;**12**:S45. DOI: 10.1016/j.cardfail.2006.06.161

[22] Maradey JA, Singleton M, Neill TJ, Bhave P. Management of ventricular

arrhythmias in patients with LVAD. Current Opinion in Cardiology. 2020;**35**:289-294

[23] Kociol RD. Time for MADIT-VAD? JACC: Heart Failure. octubre de. 2016;**4**(10):780-782. DOI: 10.1016/j.jchf.2016.08.003

[24] Oz MC, Rose EA, Slater J, Kuiper JJ, Catanese KA, Levin HR. Malignant ventricular dysrhythmias are well tolerated in patients receiving long-term left ventricular assist devices. Journal of the American College of Cardiology. 1994;**24**:1688-1691. DOI: 10.1016/0735-1097(94)90175-9

[25] Sims DB, Rosner G, Uriel N, González-Costello J, Ehlert FA, Jorde UP. Twelve hours of sustained ventricular fibrillation supported by a continuous-flow left ventricular assist device. Pacing and Clinical Electrophysiology. 2012;**35**:e144-e148

[26] Busch MC, Haap M, Kristen A, Haas CS. Asymptomatic sustained ventricular fibrillation in a patient with left ventricular assist device. Annals of Emergency Medicine. 2011;**57**(1):25-28. DOI: 10.1016/j.annemergmed.2010.05.023

[27] Smith ME, Moak JH. Asymptomatic ventricular fibrillation in continuous flow left-ventricular assist device. The American Journal of Emergency Medicine. 2021;**49**:130-132. DOI: 10.1016/j.ajem.2021.05.065

[28] Clerkin KJ, Topkara VK, Demmer RT, Dizon JM, Yuzefpolskaya M, Fried JA, et al. Implantable cardioverter defibrillators in patients with a continuous-flow left ventricular assist device: An Analysis of the INTERMACS Registry. JACC Heart Fail. diciembre de. 2017;**5**(12):916-926. DOI: 10.1016/j.jchf.2017.08.014

[29] Rorris FP, Antonopoulos CN, Kyriakopoulos CP, Drakos SG, Charitos C. Implantable cardioverter defibrillators in left ventricular assist device patients: A systematic review and meta-analysis. Journal of Heart and Lung Transplantation. 2021;**40**(10):1098-1106. DOI: 10.1016/j.healun.2021.05.014

[30] Kutyifa V, Fernandez G, Sherazi S, Aktas M, Huang D, McNitt S, et al. Implantable cardioverter defibrillators and survival in continuous-flow left ventricular assist device patients. ASAIO Journal. 2019;**65**(1):49-53. DOI: 10.1097/MAT.0000000000000739

[31] Younes A, Al-Kindi SG, Alajaji W, Mackall JA, Oliveira GH. Presence of implantable cardioverter-defibrillators and wait-list mortality of patients supported with left ventricular assist devices as a bridge to heart transplantation. International Journal of Cardiology. 2017;**231**:211-215. DOI: 10.1016/j.ijcard.2016.12.148

[32] Riaz T, Nienaber JJ, Baddour LM, et al. Cardiovascular implantable electronic device infections in left ventricular assist device recipients. Pacing and Clinical Electrophysiology. 2014;**37**(2):225-230. DOI: 10.1111/pace.12240

[33] Schron EB, Exner DV, Yao Q, et al. Quality of life in the antiarrhythmics versus implantable defibrillators trial: Impact of therapy and influence of adverse symptoms and defibrillator shocks. Circulation. 2002;**105**(5):589-594. DOI: 10.1161/hc0502.103330

[34] Potapov EV, Antonides C, Crespo-Leiro MG, Combes A, Färber G, Hannan MM, et al. EACTS Expert Consensus on long-term mechanical circulatory support. European Journal of Cardio-Thoracic Surgery.

2019;**56**(2):230-270. DOI: 10.1093/ejcts/ezz098

[35] Zeppenfeld K, Tfelt-Hansen J, de Riva M, Winkel BG, Behr ER, et al. 2022 ESC Guidelines for the management of patients with ventricular dysrhythmias and the prevention of sudden cardiac death: Developed by the task force for the management of patients with ventricular dysrhythmias and the prevention of sudden cardiac death of the European Society of Cardiology (ESC) Endorsed by the Association for European Paediatric and Congenital Cardiology (AEPC). European Heart Journal. 2022;**2022**:262

[36] Cikes M, Jakus N, Claggett B, Brugts JJ, Timmermans P, Pouleur A-C, et al. Cardiac implantable electronic devices with a defibrillator component and all-cause mortality in left ventricular assist device carriers: Results from the PCHF-VAD registry. European Journal of Heart Failure. 2019;**21**:1129-1141. DOI: 10.1002/ejhf.1568

[37] Galand V, Fléсher E, Auffret V, Boulé S, Vincentelli A, Dambrin C, et al. Predictors and clinical impact of late ventricular dysrhythmias in patients with continuous-flow left ventricular assist devices. JACC Clinical Electrophysiology. 2018;**4**:1166-1175. DOI: 10.1016/j.jacep.2018.05.006

[38] Kutyifa V, Moss AJ, Schuger C, Mcnitt S, Polonsky B, Ruwald ACH, et al. Reduction in inappropriate ICD therapy in MADIT-RIT patients without history of atrial tachyarrhythmia. Journal of Cardiovascular Electrophysiology. 2015;**26**(8):879-884. DOI: 10.1111/jce.12692

[39] Gasparini M, Proclemer A, Klersy C, et al. Effect of long-detection interval vs standard-detection interval for implantable cardioverter-defibrillators on anti-tachycardia pacing and shock delivery: The advance iii randomized clinical trial. Journal of the American Medical Association. 2013;**309**:1903-1911. DOI: 10.1001/jama.2013.4598

[40] Schleifer JW, Mookadam F, Kransdorf EP, Nanda U, Adams JC, Cha S, et al. Effect of continued cardiac resynchronization therapy on ventricular dysrhythmias after left ventricular assist device implantation. American Journal of Cardiology. 2016;**118**:556-559

[41] Gopinathannair R, Birks EJ, Trivedi JR, McCants KC, Sutton BS, Deam AG, et al. Impact of cardiac resynchronization therapy on clinical outcomes in patients with continuous-flow left ventricular assist devices. Journal of Cardiac Failure. 2015;**21**:226-232. DOI: 10.1016/j.cardfail.2014.12.006

[42] Muratsu J, Hara M, Mizote I, Asano Y, Sakata Y, Saito S, et al. The impact of cardiac resynchronization therapy in an end-stage heart failure patient with a left ventricular assist device as a bridge to recovery. A case report. International Heart Journal. 2011;**52**(4):246-247. DOI: 10.1536/ihj.52.246

[43] Schnegg B, Robson D, Fürholz M, Meredith T, Kessler C, Baldinger SH, et al. Importance of electromagnetic interactions between ICD and VAD devices-Mechanistic assessment. Artificial Organs. 2022;**46**(6):1132-1141. DOI: 10.1111/aor.14167

[44] Abbot. Reported ICD Experience with the HeartMate 3 LVAD [Internet]. 2022. Available from: https://www.cardiovascular.abbott/us/en/hcp/products/heart-failure/left-ventricular-assist-devices/heartmate-3/indications-safety-warnings/heartmate-3-reported-icd-experience.html [Accessed: June 28, 2022]

[45] Yalcin YC, Kooij C, Theuns DAMJ, Constantinescu AA, Brugts JJ,

Manintveld OC, et al. Emerging electromagnetic interferences between implantable cardioverter-defibrillators and left ventricular assist devices. EP Europace. 2020;**22**(4):584-587

[46] Foo D, Walker BD, Kuchar DL, Thorburn CW, Tay A, Hayward CS, et al. Left ventricular mechanical assist devices and cardiac device interactions: An observational case series. Pacing and Clinical Electrophysiology. 2009;**32**: 879-887. DOI: 10.1111/j.1540-8159.2009.02403.x

[47] Khetarpal BK, Lee JZ, Javaid AI, Srivathsan KS. B-PO05-063 Heartware left ventricular assist device associated telemetry interference and lead noise in transvenous implantable cardioverter-defibrillators. Heart Rhythm. 2021;**18**(8):S397

[48] Ambardekar AV, Lowery CM, Allen LA, Cannon AP, Cleveland JC Jr, Lindenfeld J, et al. Effect of left ventricular assist device placement on preexisting implantable cardioverter-defibrillator leads. Journal of Cardiac Failure. 2010;**16**:327-331. DOI: 10.1016/j.cardfail.2009.12.003

[49] Kühne M, Sakumura M, Reich SS, Sarrazin JF, Wells D, Chalfoun N, et al. Simultaneous use of implantable cardioverter-defibrillators and left ventricular assist devices in patients with severe heart failure. The American Journal of Cardiology. 2010;**105**(3):378-382

[50] Black-Maier E, Lewis RK, Barnett AS, Pokorney SD, Sun AY, Koontz JI, et al. Subcutaneous implantable cardioverter-defibrillator troubleshooting in patients with a left ventricular assist device: A case series and systematic review. Heart Rhythm. 2020;**17**(9):1536-1544

[51] López-Gil M, Fontenla A, Delgado JF, Rodríguez-Muñoz D. Subcutaneous implantable cardioverter defibrillators in patients with left ventricular assist devices: Case report and comprehensive review. European Heart Journal of Case Report. 2019;**3**(2):ytz057

Section 4

Management of Complications during Mechanical Circulatory Support

Chapter 5

Recurrent Heart Failure after Left Ventricular Assist Device Placement

Tamas Alexy and Michael A. Burke

Abstract

A host of complications are common after left ventricular assist device (LVAD) surgery. Perhaps none is more challenging to manage than recurrent heart failure (HF). HF in an LVAD patient is associated with substantial morbidity and increased mortality. HF can occur early or late, can present abruptly or insidiously, and can be due to an array of LVAD-specific problems including pump thrombosis and cannula obstruction, or intrinsic cardiac problems such as right ventricular failure or valvular disease. These disparate etiologies require specific testing and distinct therapeutic strategies. This chapter reviews the causes of recurrent HF after LVAD surgery with particular attention to evaluation and management strategies that can identify and treat these distinct etiologies.

Keywords: LVAD, recurrent heart failure, right heart failure, outflow graft obstruction, valvular heart disease

1. Introduction

Heart failure (HF) is among the commonest chronic diseases, with a prevalence of 6.2 million adults in the United States (U.S.) and 64.3 million worldwide [1, 2]. Patients with the most advanced form of HF are classified as stage D and have high mortality. Population studies estimate the prevalence of stage D HF to be between 0.2–3.0% [3], with up to 4.5% of patients with chronic (stage C) HF progressing to stage D per year [4]. In the U.S., this is ~150,000–250,000 with stage D disease [3, 5]. Orthotopic heart transplantation (OHT) remains the gold standard therapy for this population. However, there remains a tremendous shortfall of available organs; despite recent increases, only 3817 OHT surgeries were performed in the U.S. in 2021 (~1.5–2.5% of the estimated stage D population) [6].

Left ventricular assist device (LVAD) surgery has revolutionized the treatment of end-stage HF, providing increased longevity and a superior quality of life (QOL) for patients with stage D disease. LVAD technology has progressed dramatically over the last 3 decades, with each successive generation of pump providing robust improvements in outcomes [7]. However, LVAD-associated morbidity remains substantial (**Figure 1**) [8, 9]. Among the commonest complications is recurrent HF. This is almost uniformly associated with increased mortality and worse QOL.

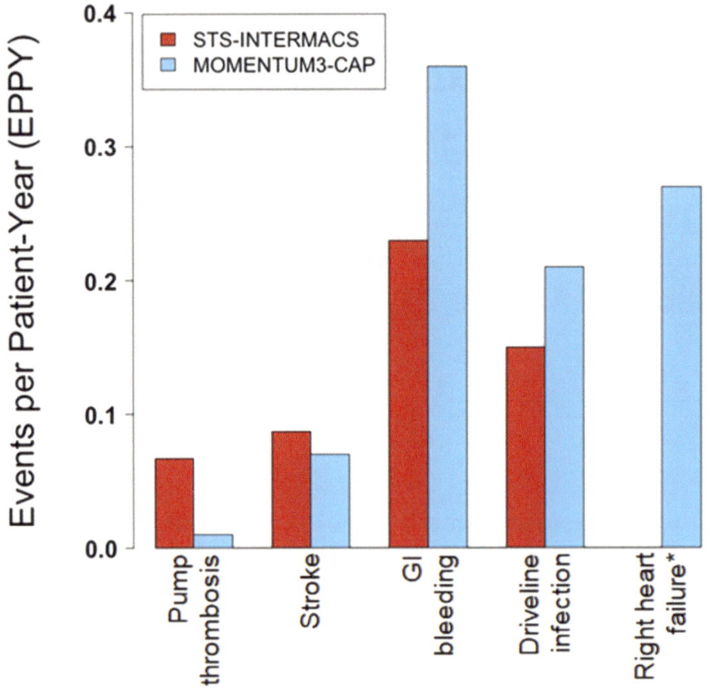

Figure 1.
*Contemporary adverse event rates after LVAD. Events per patient-year (EEPY) occurring >90 days after implant in the STS-INTERMACS registry [8], or from the MOMENTUM 3 continued access protocol (CAP) trial [9]. *No event rate data exist for right HF from STS-INTERMACS.*

Recurrent HF after LVAD has many causes and critically, management depends on the underlying etiology. Recurrent HF is either related to problems extrinsic to the LVAD or to a problem with the device itself (**Figure 2**) [10]. By far the commonest cause is failure of the right ventricle (RV). This chapter will review the causes of recurrent HF and provide strategies to diagnose and manage these distinct problems.

2. Causes of recurrent heart failure

2.1 Right heart failure

2.1.1 Defining right heart failure

Failure of the RV is the commonest cause of recurrent HF after LVAD surgery. The reported prevalence of RV failure is extremely variable, ranging from 4 to 40% for continuous flow devices [11]. This variance is driven by a lack of standardization in post-operative management, differences in patient characteristics between implanting centers, and the wide range in follow-up time across studies.

The evolution of LVAD technology and usage have impacted the prevalence of RV failure. Though the pulsatile HeartMate XVE was approved for use as destination therapy (DT) in 2003, 2-year survival was low (23% in the REMATCH trial [12], 33% in a post-REMATCH registry [13], and 24% in the HeartMate II (HMII)

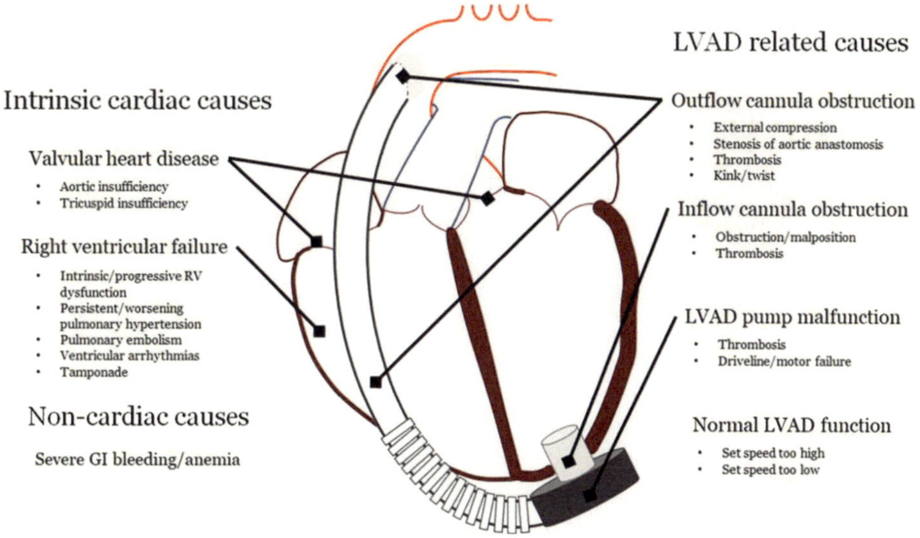

Figure 2.
Causes of recurrent heart failure (HF) after LVAD implant. HF can be caused by intrinsic cardiac disease that is pre-existing or that develops after LVAD implant, or may be secondary to severe anemia in the setting of GI bleeding. Alternately, HF may result from LVAD-specific issues, including outflow or inflow cannula obstruction, pump failure, or simply an inappropriate LVAD set speed.

DT trial [14]) owing at least in part to mechanical failure of this pump. Further, the size of the HeartMate XVE restricted its use to larger patients. These factors limited long-term use, and bridge-to-transplantation (BTT) remained the dominant implant strategy in the first decade of the 2000s [15]. Consequently, analyses of HF in LVAD patients from >10 years ago largely focused on early post-operative RV failure. However, since approval of the HMII for DT in January 2010, DT has become the dominant implant strategy in the U.S. (**Figure 3**) [16]. This has led to substantially longer time on LVAD support with a concomitant shift in patient characteristics and outcomes. Finally, changes to the United Network for Organ Sharing OHT listing criteria in 2018 and advances in the use of temporary mechanical circulatory support (MCS), have resulted in an even more significant reduction in BTT LVAD usage in the last 3 years [17].

Analysis of recurrent HF has also been hampered by the variable definitions used for RV failure. Nearly all studies define RV failure when a right ventricular assist device (RVAD) is required, but inotrope use as a criterion has been variable as has the requirement for clinical signs of HF. In 2008, the Interagency Registry for Mechanically Assisted Circulatory Support (INTERMACS) defined RV failure by a central venous pressure (CVP) >18 mmHg, cardiac index <2.0 L/min/m^2 and either the need for an RVAD, or any use of vasoactive medications >7 days after LVAD implant. The limitations of this definition were quickly recognized, and it was revised in 2014 (**Table 1**). This refined definition required (1) elevated right sided filling pressures and (2) physical or laboratory evidence for congestion. If these criteria were met, then the severity of RV failure was further qualified.

Though the 2014 definition was more inclusive, some patients with RV failure were still not captured, and hybrid definitions remained commonplace. In 2020, the Academic Research Consortium convened a multidisciplinary working group to

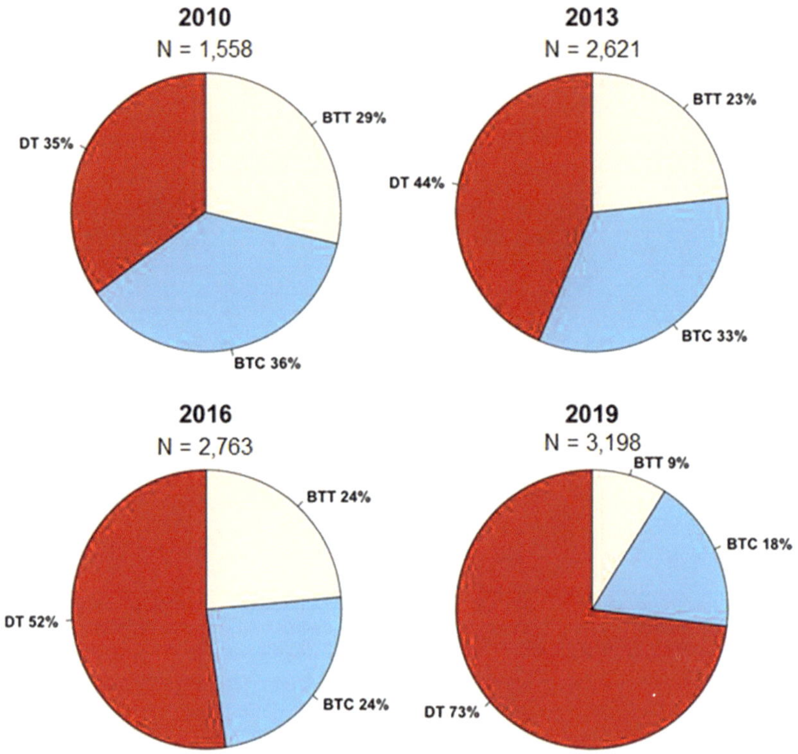

Figure 3.
Evolution of continuous flow LVAD implant strategies in the U.S. (2010–2019). The total number of implants per year is listed below each year. From: STS-INTERMACS database [16].

define adverse events related to MCS use (MCS-ARC) [18]. In this simplified definition, RV failure is divided into early or late based on the timing relative to LVAD surgery (**Table 2**). The need for an RVAD continues to define right HF, while vasoactive medication use without RVAD requires that additional clinical criteria be met including findings of elevated right atrial pressure, or evidence of end organ dysfunction/hypoperfusion. In late 2021, the Society of Thoracic Surgeons (STS)-INTERMACS database adopted this MCS-ARC definition of right HF [19].

2.1.2 Right heart function in the LVAD patient

The RV is anatomically and physiologically distinct from the LV [20]. Under normal conditions, RV output is roughly equal to that of the LV. However, the mechanics of RV contraction are distinct. The RV is thin walled and shaped like a tetrahedron (**Figure 4**). It is highly compliant and pumps blood into the low impedance pulmonary vasculature. Consequently, the RV requires only one sixth the energy of the LV per contraction [20]. As the LV contracts, it twists around its longitudinal axis; this twisting motion (akin to wringing a wet towel) contributes significantly to septal contraction. Meanwhile the RV contracts along longitudinal and transverse axes, with longitudinal shortening being the major driver of RV stroke volume (**Figure 5**) [21]. Importantly, a significant portion of longitudinal RV contractility is derived from the septum.

Part 1: Symptoms or findings of right heart failure (need to meet both)	
Documented elevation of CVP	1. Directly measured right atrial pressure > 16 mmHg — OR — IVC with absence of inspiratory variation by echocardiography — OR — 3. elevated JVP halfway up neck in an upright patient
Manifestations of systemic venous congestion	1. Peripheral edema — OR — 2. Ascites ± palpable hepatomegaly — OR — 3. Laboratory evidence: serum creatinine >2 mg/dL or total bilirubin >2.0 mg/dL
Part 2: If patient meets the definition for right heart failure (Part 1), then severity is classified as:	
Mild	Vasoactive meds (inotropes, vasopressors, vasodilators) are not continued for >7 days post-LVAD implant
Moderate	Vasoactive meds (inotropes, vasopressors, vasodilators) are required for >7 but ≤14 days post-LVAD implant
Severe	Vasoactive meds (inotropes, vasopressors, vasodilators) are required >14 days post-LVAD implant — AND — Persistently elevated CVP >16 mmHg
Severe acute	Need for RVAD support at any time following LVAD implant — OR — Death during the LVAD implant hospitalization with right heart failure as the primary cause

CVP – central venous pressure; IVC – inferior vena cava; JVP – jugular venous pressure; RVAD – right ventricular assist device.

Table 1.
2014 INTERMACS definition of right heart failure.

RV function is primarily governed by three physiologic parameters: (1) preload; (2) contractility; and (3) afterload. In chronic HF, primary RV dysfunction (i.e., independent of LV failure) is common, being identified in about half of patients with HF and reduced ejection fraction [22]. RV afterload is determined by pulmonary vascular resistance (PVR) and compliance. The RV displays a steep decline in cardiac output with increasing PVR [20]. In chronic HF, PVR rises and compliance declines secondary to (1) elevated left heart pressures and (2) pulmonary arterial remodeling, thus substantially increasing RV afterload.

Right HF after LVAD implant is multifactorial. The abrupt increase in venous return to the right heart can cause HF in a myopathic RV that fails to adequately compensate for the increased preload. RV contractility can be compromised by LVAD support in multiple ways (**Figure 5**): (1) reduced LV preload leads to a leftward shift of the septum, limiting the contribution of septal contraction to RV force generation; (2) apical LVAD insertion coupled with the loss of pericardial constraint reduces LV contractility (especially twisting), which also limits septal contraction; and (3) the leftward shift of the septum can lead to stretching of the tricuspid valve (TV)

Early acute right heart failure	Need for RVAD support (temporary or durable) during the LVAD implant operation
Early post-implant right heart failure	1. Need for RVAD support (temporary or durable) <30 days following LVAD implant — OR — 2. Failure to wean vasoactive medication (inotropes, vasopressors or inhaled pulmonary vasodilators) ≤14 days following LVAD implant OR initiation of vasoactive medication support ≤30 days of LVAD implant for a duration of ≥14 days PLUS 2 clinical findings* or 1 manifestation† of RV failure
Late right heart failure	1. Need for RVAD support (temporary or durable) >30 days following LVAD implant — OR — 2. Hospitalization >30 days following LVAD implant and which requires IV diuretics and/or inotropic support for ≥72 hours PLUS 2 clinical findings* or 1 manifestation† of RV failure

**Clinical findings of RV failure: (1) ascites; (2) functional/limiting peripheral edema; (3) elevated JVP halfway up the neck in an upright patient; (4) measured CVP >16 mmHg.*
†Manifestations of RV failure: (1) serum creatinine >2 times baseline; (2) ALT/AST ≥2 times the upper limit of normal or total serum bilirubin >2.0 mg/dL; (3) reduction in LVAD pump flow >30% below baseline in the absence of cardiac tamponade; (4) central or mixed venous blood oxygen <50%; (5) cardiac index <2.2 L/min/m2; (6) serum lactate >3.0 mmol/L.

Table 2.
2020 MCS-ARC & 2021 STS-INTERMACS definition of right heart failure.

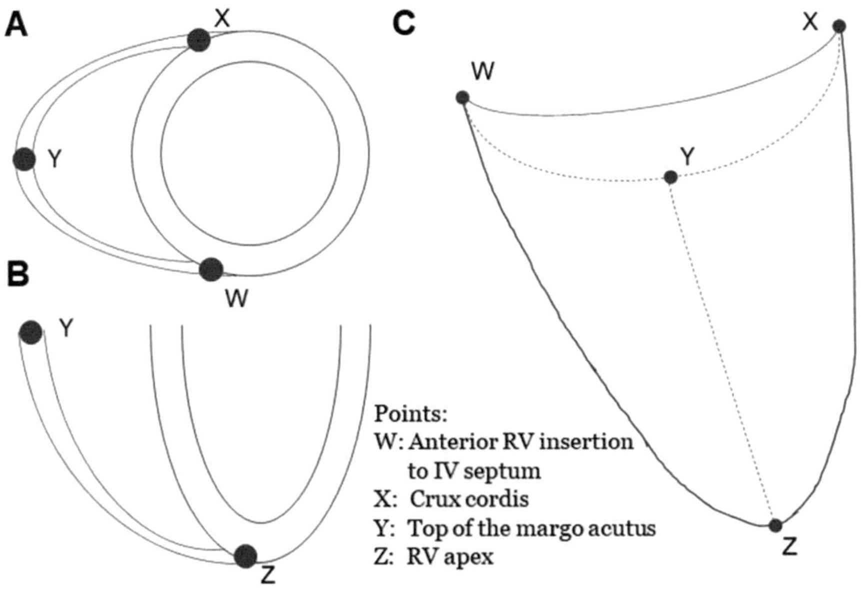

Figure 4.
*Anatomy and geometry of the right ventricle. Transverse (**A**), coronal (**B**) and sagittal (**C**) views of the heart showing the unique tetrahedral or half-ellipsoid shape of the RV. The sagittal view (**C**) is from the perspective of the interventricular (IV) septum in the foreground and looking "into" the RV towards the RV free wall. Lines correspond to the following: WX = junction of the interatrial and IV septa; WY = anterior atrioventricular sulcus; XZ = posterior atrioventricular sulcus; WZ = anterior IV sulcus; XZ = posterior IV sulcus; YZ = margo acutus. RV regions correspond to the following: WXY = approximate valvualr plane; WYZ = anterior RV free wall; XYZ = posterior RV free wall; WXZ = IV septum.*

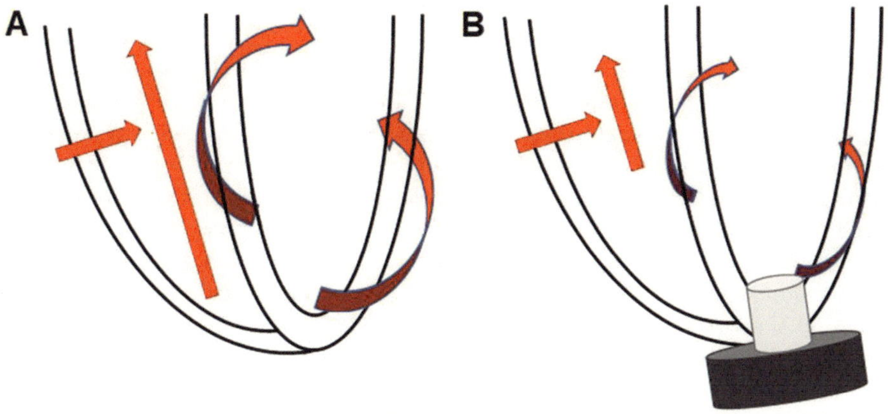

Figure 5.
*Vectors of ventricular contraction. (**A**) In the normal heart, the LV contracts in a wringing, or spiral, motion around its long axis while the normal RV contracts in perpendicular planes along its longitudinal and transverse axes. This LV twisting motion augments septal contractility and RV stroke volume. (B) An LVAD limits LV twisting and triggers a leftward shift of the interventricular septum by decreasing LV preload, in turn reducing septal contraction and overall RV longitudinal contractility. If RV free wall contractility cannot increase to compensate, then total RV cardiac output may decline.*

annulus with a concomitant increase in tricuspid regurgitation (TR). Finally, the abrupt reduction in left heart filling pressures after LVAD typically improves PVR, reducing RV afterload and improving contractility [23]. However, PVR (and therefore RV afterload) may remain elevated due to vascular remodeling, thus further contributing to post-LVAD RV failure.

2.1.3 Early right heart failure

Early right HF increases the risk of death and end-organ dysfunction, prolongs hospital length-of-stay (LOS), delays recovery, and reduces functional capacity [24–26]. The most consistent defining feature of early right HF is the need for RVAD support. In clinical trials, early RVAD support has been steady: HMII BTT trial, 6%; [27] ADVANCE trial of the HeartWare LVAD (HVAD), 2.1%; [28] MOMENTUM 3 trial of the HM3, 4.1% [9]. Registry data have shown a similar prevalence of RVAD use in patients with continuous flow LVADs: INTERMACS, 4.1%; [8] EUROMACS 2017–2020 cohort (European Registry for Patients with Mechanical Circulatory Support), 5.4%; [29] IMACS (ISHLT Mechanically Assisted Circulatory Support registry), 6.1%; [30] and MOMENTUM 3 continued access protocol (CAP) registry, 7.6% [9].

However, the reported prevalence of all early right HF events has been plagued by variable definitions. In the HMII BTT trial, early right HF was defined as the need for RVAD or inotrope support for at least 14 days following LVAD implant [27]. Using this definition, 13% had early right HF. In the HMII DT trial, early right HF was identified in 17.5%, with 43% of those with early right HF dying within 30 days of LVAD surgery [31]. In the ADVANCE trial, 14.3% were diagnosed with early right HF [28]. The prevalence of early right HF was 25% in a meta-analysis of 36 studies (4428 LVADs), however differences were noted in study design, right HF definition, and proportion of continuous flow devices [32]. In the INTERMACS database, the prevalence of right HF 1 month after LVAD implant was 24% [33]. Notably, right HF resolved in 96.5% of these individuals by 12 months. Similarly, in EUROMACS, the prevalence of early right HF was 21.7% [34].

Peri-operative factors contribute significantly to early right HF. Most LVADs are implanted with cardiopulmonary bypass (CPB) support. While CPB maintains adequate organ perfusion and gas exchange, blood contact with the circuit provokes an inflammatory response that leads to increased capillary permeability, vasoplegia, and acute organ dysfunction [35, 36]. The large volume of priming solution administered upon CPB initiation may cause volume overload and RV dysfunction [37]. Blood loss, platelet dysfunction and coagulopathy often mandate transfusion, which can also contribute to right HF [38]. Finally, myocardial stunning [39], pericardiotomy-associated changes in RV contraction [40, 41], pulmonary hypertension [42], and inadvertent air embolism to the right coronary artery [43] may all contribute to acute RV dysfunction.

2.1.4 Late right heart failure

Even more than early right HF, analysis of late right HF has been plagued by variable definitions, different clinical parameters (e.g., time from surgery, type of support, presence of HF symptoms) and study types (e.g., single-center, clinical trials) that may not be representative of the general LVAD population [44]. Study duration is also critical: 59% of right HF was diagnosed >1 year after LVAD implant in the HMII DT trial [31], and de novo late right HF in the STS-INTERMACS database developed at a relatively constant rate of 5–10% [33, 45].

In the HMII BTT trial, late right HF was defined as initiation of inotropes >14 days after implant. Using this simplistic definition, 7% had late RV failure [27]. However, the median duration on LVAD support was only 126 days [46]. In the HMII DT trial, RV failure occurred in 21% over a median follow-up of 1.7 years at a rate of 0.13 events per patient-year (EPPY) [47]. When divided into early and late right HF (causing hospitalization >30 days post-LVAD), late right HF was identified in 8% of DT patients at a median of 480 days after LVAD implant [31].

In the ADVANCE trial, inotropes were used beyond 30 days in 6% (0.12 EPPY) [28]. Longer follow-up from the HVAD registry found RV failure in 9% (0.10 EPPY), though events were not adjudicated as early or late [48]. Similarly, the MOMENTUM 3 trial did not split early from late right HF events, simply defining RV failure as "symptoms and signs" of RV dysfunction with either RVAD implant, or therapy with inhaled nitric oxide or inotropes for >1 week at any point after LVAD surgery [49]. In MOMENTUM 3-CAP, right HF (early and late) was identified in ~37% (0.27 EPPY) [9].

In the National Readmission Database, 4.2% of all patients discharged after the implant hospitalization were readmitted with recurrent HF within 30 days of discharge (13.4% of all readmissions) [50]. When using the 2014 INTERMACS definition (**Table 1**) in patients who survived 3 months after LVAD surgery, the incidence of new, mild RV failure was 5–6% at 12-months, with moderate HF in an additional 4–5%, and severe HF being very rare as a late presentation (≤0.2%). In a single center study of DT patients who survived 1-year post-LVAD surgery without right HF, 45% developed right HF at a steady rate over a mean of 3.5 years [51]. Importantly, this incidence of de novo right HF, while highest in the early post-op period, appears to stabilize at 5–10% by 3–6 months post-LVAD implant and remains steady for at least 4–5 years [33, 45, 51, 52].

The prevalence of right HF after LVAD implant is ~10% by 3 months and remains constant for ≥3 years [33]. After diagnosis of late right HF, 9–20% will die and an additional ~25–33% will have persistent HF within 3–6 months [33, 45]. Two factors seem to predict persistence of RV failure. First is the time from LVAD implant to diagnosis of right HF, with HF that develops later associated with a higher rate of persistence [33]. Second is the severity of HF at diagnosis: of patients with no right HF 3 months post-LVAD, only 3.4% developed HF at 6- or 12-months after surgery. By contrast, of those with moderate right HF 3 months after implant, HF persisted in 32.5% and 11.5% at 6- and 12-months, respectively [45].

2.1.5 Outcomes associated with right heart failure

Right HF is a morbid complication in LVAD patients; this includes increased rehospitalizations, excess complications, poorer functional metrics and, critically, worse survival. Right HF has been adjudicated as the cause of death in 11–13% in the STS-INTERMACS [8] and IMACS registries [30]. Right HF as the cause of death in clinical trials has been more variable: 5% for continuous flow devices in the HMII DT trial [14], 12% in the ROADMAP trial (also HMII) [53], 17% in the ADVANCE trial (HVAD) [28], and 28% in the MOMENTUM 3 trial (HM3) [7].

In the HMII BTT trial, early RV failure was associated with a lower combined end point of (1) survival to OHT, (2) recovery, or (3) continuing support at 180 days (71% vs. 89% without right HF; $p < 0.001$); those requiring an RVAD had the poorest outcomes [27]. In a single high-volume center, 6-month mortality with early RVAD use was 41% [54]. This study also showed that (1) successful RVAD weaning was associated with ~3-fold better survival; and (2) planned biventricular support during the index surgery yielded better outcomes than later RVAD implant. A meta-analysis of retrospective studies found that RVAD use after LVAD was associated with significantly worse survival, and increased rates of bleeding and stroke [55]. Finally, data from INTERMACS [24] and EUROMACS [56] show that RVAD use is associated with lower 1-month, 6-month and 1-year survival.

Late right HF is also associated with reduced survival [31, 45, 57]. In the HMII DT trial, patients with late right HF had lower 1-year (78% vs. 84%), 2-year (58% vs. 81%) and 3-year survival (36% vs. 56%, $p < 0.001$) [31]. Notably, when analyzed from the time of diagnosis of de novo right HF, 1-year survival in this DT cohort was only 38%. BTT patients have reduced survival to OHT if right HF develops. In STS-INTERMACS, the presence and severity of late right HF predicted worse outcomes, including mortality (**Figure 6**) [45]. Perhaps not surprisingly, those with persistent right HF have the worst outcomes [33]. Finally, late right HF was associated with modest but significantly more strokes, arrhythmias and infections [45]. However, a causal link to right HF has not been established.

Post-LVAD right HF may also put patients at elevated risk after OHT. Patients requiring an RVAD with a BTT LVAD had a 22% increase risk of death post-OHT [58]. A retrospective, large, single-center study showed reduced post-OHT survival up to 5-years in BTT LVAD patients who developed right HF [57]. A study of 2 large European transplant centers found a post-OHT 1-year survival of 75% in BTT LVAD patients with right HF; [59] while not significant in their cohort, this is substantially lower than the ~93% 1-year post-OHT survival in the International Thoracic Organ Transplant Registry [60]. The mechanism for this risk is not clear. BTT LVAD use increases the risk for primary graft dysfunction (PGD) [61], and 2 single center analyses found an increased risk for PGD in BTT patients with pre-OHT right HF [57, 62].

Finally, right HF after LVAD has a negative impact on functional capacity and possibly QOL. Early RVAD use is associated with poorer QOL in some patients [63]. In the HMII DT trial, those with late right HF had lower QOL as assessed by the

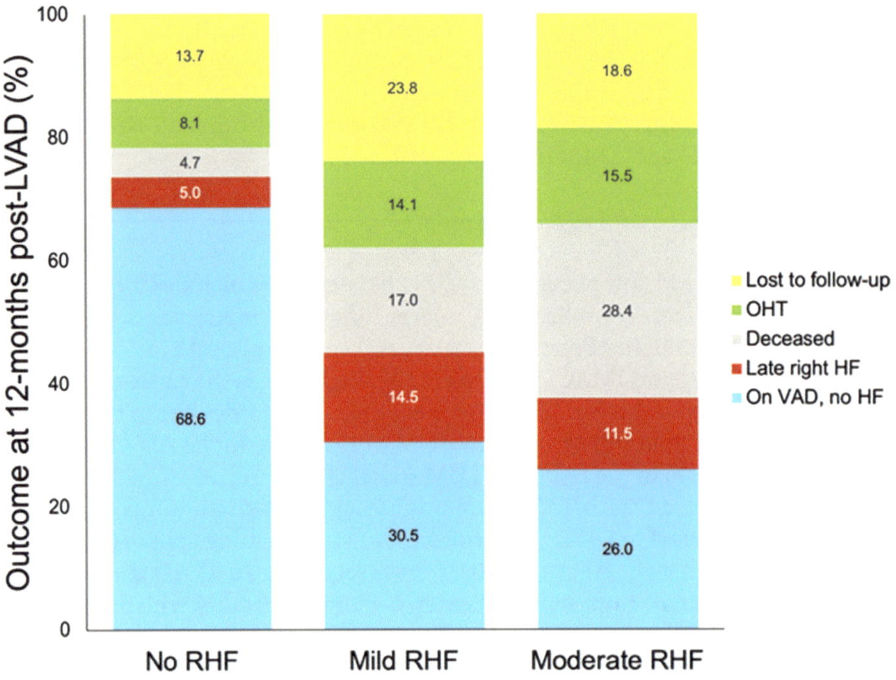

Figure 6.
Clinical outcome at 12-months in patients who survived to 3-months after LVAD implant. Patients are grouped by right heart failure (RHF) status 3-months post-LVAD. From: STS-INTERMACS database [45].

Kansas City Cardiomyopathy Questionnaire [31]. This was not true of patients in STS-INTERMACS using a visual acuity scale; [45] these investigators noted ample missing data that could have biased the analysis, and a lack of agreement as to the optimal tool for assessing QOL in LVAD patients. Functionally, those with right HF have a reduced 6-minute walk distance, supporting a detrimental effect of recurrent HF in LVAD patients [31, 45, 64, 65].

2.1.6 Predicting right heart failure after LVAD surgery

Numerous attempts have been made to predict post-LVAD RV failure in order to better guide patient selection and improve post-operative outcomes. Close to 100 variables have been found to be associated with post-LVAD right HF across dozens of studies [11, 66]. A handful of these risk factors have been consistently identified in multiple studies (**Table 3**). Although some variables are not actionable, others can be mitigated. While these predictors generally have high specificity, their sensitivity and negative predictive value are low, limiting their utility in clinical practice. A meta-analysis found that no single parameter was sufficiently sensitive to predict post-LVAD right HF [32].

Scoring systems have been developed that use a combination of these risk factors to predict post-LVAD right HF. More than 20 such models exist, most from single-center cohorts [11]. Fewer than 40% have been validated in ≥2 external cohorts. The validation studies are fraught with bias and have consistently shown poor discriminatory power with C-statistics of only 0.53–0.65 [67]. Modeling has been hindered by the many variable definitions of right HF. Further, nearly all models were derived

Clinical risk factors	• Lower heart rate • Female sex • Lower body surface area • Non-ischemic etiology for heart failure • HeartWare LVAD use • LVAD implant as destination therapy • Presence of pulmonary vascular disease • Prior coronary artery bypass or valve surgery
Laboratory risk factors	• Elevated white blood cell count • Anemia (hemoglobin ≤10 g/dL), thrombocytopenia • Abnormal renal function (elevated BUN, Cr) • Abnormal liver function (ALT, AST, total bilirubin) • Elevated INR
Echocardiographic risk factors	• Qualitatively severe RV dysfunction • Reduced RV free wall longitudinal strain • Increased RV end diastolic diameter • Lower LV end diastolic diameter • Increased ratio of RV to LV diastolic area • Higher LV ejection fraction • Moderate/severe tricuspid regurgitation • Increased left atrial volume
Hemodynamic risk factors	• Low systolic blood pressure • Elevated central venous pressure (CVP) • High CVP/pulmonary capillary wedge pressure ratio • Low pulmonary artery pulsatility index • Low RV stroke work index • Elevated pulmonary vascular resistance • Cardiac index ≤2.2 L/min/m^2 • Pre-operative need for inotropes/MCS/IABP
Perioperative risk factors	• Need for mechanical ventilatory support • INTERMACS profile • Hemodialysis or ultrafiltration with 48 hours of LVAD • Circulatory support (e.g., ECMO, percutaneous VAD) • Inotrope use • Vasopressor use • Intraoperative bleeding or need for re-operation • Prolonged cardiopulmonary bypass time • Other concomitant procedure performed at the time of LVAD surgery

BUN – blood urea nitrogen; Cr – creatinine; ALT – alanine aminotransferase; AST – aspartate aminotransferase; INR – international normalized ratio; LV – left ventricle; RV – right ventricle; MCS – mechanical circulatory support; IABP – intraaortic balloon pump; ECMO – extracorporeal membrane oxygenation.

Table 3.
Risk factors for post-LVAD right heart failure.

using data from pulsatile or early-generation continuous flow LVADs, limiting their applicability. Consequently, results have been disappointing, and have limited wider use of these predictive models in clinical practice.

2.2 Valvular heart disease

2.2.1 Aortic regurgitation

Significant aortic valve insufficiency (AI) can create a short circulation loop in LVAD patients whereby a substantial fraction of the blood pumped by the LVAD to the aorta returns directly to the LV (**Figure 7**). This reduces effective perfusion, causes LV distention and elevates left heart filling pressures, ultimately causing HF. Consequently, moderate to severe AI is a contraindication to LVAD unless valve intervention is planned at the time of surgery [68].

Among patients in the STS-INTERMACS database implanted between 2016 and 2020, only 0.7% had severe AI at the time of LVAD surgery [8]. Moderate or severe AI was present at implant in 4.5% of over 16,000 patients in the IMACS database [30]. By contrast, mild AI prior to LVAD is relatively common, being found in 29.7% of patients in INTERMACS [69] and 31.2% in IMACS [70].

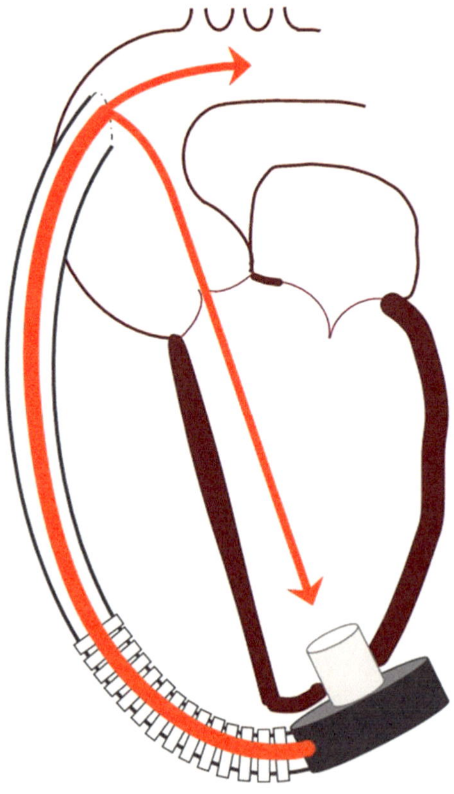

Figure 7.
Aortic valve insufficiency (AI) with an LVAD. Significant AI creates a short circulation loop whereby a substantial portion of LVAD flow regurgitates back into the LV. This reduces functional cardiac output and increases left heart filling pressures, ultimately causing heart failure.

Importantly, AI can progress or develop de novo after LVAD implant; this is clearly a result of LVAD support rather than disease progression (**Figure 8A**) [71]. Two mechanisms drive the development of AI on LVAD support. First, full LVAD support substantially reduces or completely eliminates aortic valve (AV) opening during systole. This promotes fusion of the commissures between valve leaflets; the resulting fibrosis causes retraction of the leaflets and AI with a central regurgitant jet. Second, decompression of the LV and the high volume delivered to the proximal ascending aorta generates a substantial and continuous pressure gradient across the valve that favors flow into the LV.

The prevalence of AI increases with the duration of LVAD support (**Figure 8B**); in INTERMACS, 13.2% developed moderate/severe AI over a mean follow-up of 13.4 months [69]. Of those with no AI prior to LVAD, 10.7% developed moderate or severe AI, while 18.9% with mild AI prior to LVAD developed moderate or severe AI. By 6-months post-LVAD, 55% had developed at least mild AI.

Key factors that increase the risk of significant AI across multiple studies are (1) older age at LVAD implant; (2) female sex; (3) low body surface area; (4) longer duration of LVAD support; (5) baseline mild (vs. no) AI; (6) no AV opening; and (7) continuous flow (vs. pulsatile) pump [69, 71–73]. The presence of moderate or severe AI is associated with a modest but significant increase in hospitalizations [69]. Moderate/severe AI is also associated with greater severity of MR, but surprisingly, is not associated with significantly worse QOL or reduced 6-minute walk distance. Finally, the presence of moderate or severe AI (vs. no or mild AI) is associated with lower survival (49.1% vs. 35.6% at 5-years, $p < 0.001$) [69].

2.2.2 Mitral regurgitation

Hemodynamically significant mitral regurgitation (MR) is the commonest valve lesion at the time of LVAD implant. It is almost always functional MR secondary to LV dilation. Among >26,000 patients in STS-INTERMACS, 22.8% had severe MR

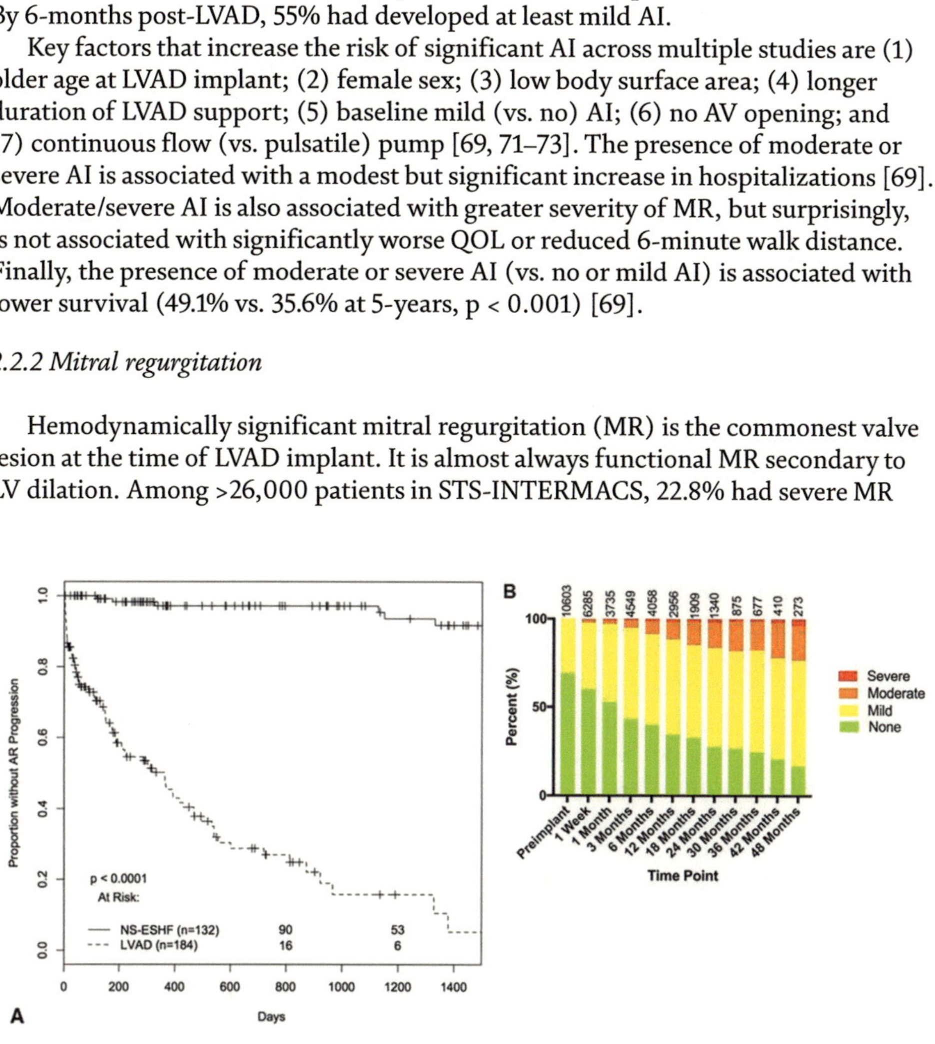

Figure 8.
*Natural history of aortic insufficiency (AI) after LVAD implant. (**A**) Proportion of patients with progression of AI from baseline up to 4-years in those receiving an LVAD as compared to patients with end-stage HF who did not undergo LVAD surgery (NS-ESHF). Reprinted with permission [71]. (**B**) Progression and severity of AI in LVAD patients from the INTERMACS database, with number of patients assessed listed above each bar. Reprinted with permission [69].*

at baseline [8]. Similarly, at implant, 57% had moderate/severe MR in IMACS [30], and 46% had moderate/severe MR, or underwent concomitant MV surgery in the MOMENTUM 3 trial [74].

With offloading of the LV, MR improves in the majority of LVAD patients [74]. When moderate to severe MR persists, the impact on outcomes remains uncertain. In the MOMENTUM 3 trial, persistent MR was uncommon (~6.5% at 1-year, n = 619), and was not associated with survival, adverse events including right HF, or functional capacity [74]. However, in INTERMACS (n = 8364), persistent MR was ~3-fold more common (18.8% at a median of 15 months), and was associated with increased rates of right HF and renal failure, and a modest 16% increase in mortality of borderline significance (p = 0.07) [75]. Single center studies also show mixed results, with frequent right HF but little to no impact on survival.

2.2.3 Tricuspid regurgitation

TR is also common in advanced HF. In the STS-INTERMACS database, 11.5% had severe TR at baseline [8], and 41% had moderate or severe TR at implant in the IMACS database [30]. Improvements in PVR and afterload with LVAD support often leads to a reduction in TR [23, 76]. Outcomes data on post-LVAD TR are very limited, but large single center studies as well as data from the EUROMACS registry suggest that moderate or severe TR after LVAD is associated with a small but significant increase in mortality [76, 77].

2.3 Device malfunction

Right HF can be caused by device malfunction, cannula obstruction or inappropriate LVAD speed. LVAD pump thrombosis is discussed elsewhere in this textbook. Data on device malfunction and outcomes are scant. Further, malfunction caused by manufacturing problems often leads to a recall, which abruptly changes incidence [78]. LVAD failure as a cause of death occurs in ~2% [8, 30], with events declining in recent years [8]. In a large single-center study, device malfunction occurred at a rate of 3.06 events per 1000 patient-days [79]. Notably, device malfunction is pump-type specific, with more events in the HMII. The only data for the HM3 comes from the European ELEVATE registry, which showed device malfunction in 3.9% [80]. However, almost 90% of these events were due to outflow graft twisting, a problem since corrected by the manufacturer.

Device malfunction can be grouped by the component that failed: (1) controller; (2) pump/driveline; and (3) peripheral components (e.g., cables, batteries, monitor). Importantly, not all malfunction results in right HF, with pump or driveline failure the most likely to result in a clinically significant event (i.e., HF or death). Controller malfunction was commonest (~30%), while pump or driveline malfunction constituted 13% of malfunction events [79].

Inflow cannula obstruction is a rare event, typically associated with thrombus and/or cannula malposition [81]. Abnormal inflow cannula position is associated with increased left heart filling pressures and a > 2-fold increased risk of recurrent HF [82]. By contrast, outflow cannula obstruction is more common and likely underappreciated; dozens of case reports and case series exist, with an event rate of 0.03 EPPY in the largest study [83]. The commonest pathology seems to be external compression from buildup of an acellular fibrinous material between the outflow graft and the protective GoreTex wrap that is frequently placed around the graft at implant.

Notably, ~80% of patients with clinically significant outflow cannula obstruction will have recurrent HF [83].

3. Management of Recurrent Heart Failure

Recurrent HF is a morbid event that limits functional capacity and survival, and therefore warrants aggressive treatment. However, management depends on the underlying etiology (**Figure 9**). Importantly, assessment of post-LVAD HF should begin prior to implant, with attention given to optimization of RV function and planning for the management of significant valvular disease at the time of surgery.

The simplest tenet of LVAD management is ensuring an appropriate LVAD speed, the only pump parameter that can be adjusted by providers. If the speed is too low, cardiac output will remain insufficient, resulting in persistent HF. By contrast, if the speed is too high, HF can result from worsening RV dysfunction (**Figure 5**) and/or worsening valve disease. Though widely used and given a Class I recommendation in the MCS guidelines [68], data supporting the utility of ramp echocardiographic studies are limited. Further, recent evidence suggests that hemodynamic-guided management by right heart catheterization may be superior to echo-guided ramp testing [84]. Ultimately, more data are needed.

3.1 Management of right heart failure

Preemptive strategies to mitigate right HF post-LVAD (whether early or late) are an essential component in management. Preoperatively, this consists of optimizing RV preload (lowering CVP), and afterload (lowering PVR and left heart filling pressures). Intraoperative strategies include judicious fluid and blood product use, and limiting time on CPB. Immediately post-LVAD, RV support with inotropes and pulmonary vasodilators is routine, as is managing vasoplegia to limit myocardial ischemia, and optimizing LVAD speed [85].

Chronic management of the LVAD patient includes maintenance of proper RV preload with diuretics, treatment of hypertension to permit optimal pump function and resumption of neurohumoral blockade, which can improve functional capacity and survival [86, 87]. Collectively these approaches are likely to limit the incidence of recurrent HF, though little data exists to support this indication. Once right HF develops, management differs depending on timing: more aggressive strategies are favored early and can frequently yield good outcomes, while late right HF usually merits a more conservative approach and has a more uniformly poor prognosis.

3.1.1 Early right heart failure

Timely identification of RV failure in the immediate postoperative period may be challenging but is of critical importance. As noted, early post-operative diuretic and inotrope use are routine. However, rising lactic acid levels, evidence of end organ dysfunction, and/or persistent or increasing vasoactive medication doses signal that RV mechanical support may be required. Importantly, the timing of RVAD initiation affects prognosis. In a multicenter retrospective analysis of 91 patients requiring RV support, an RVAD was implanted at the time of the LVAD in 44% with 56% receiving

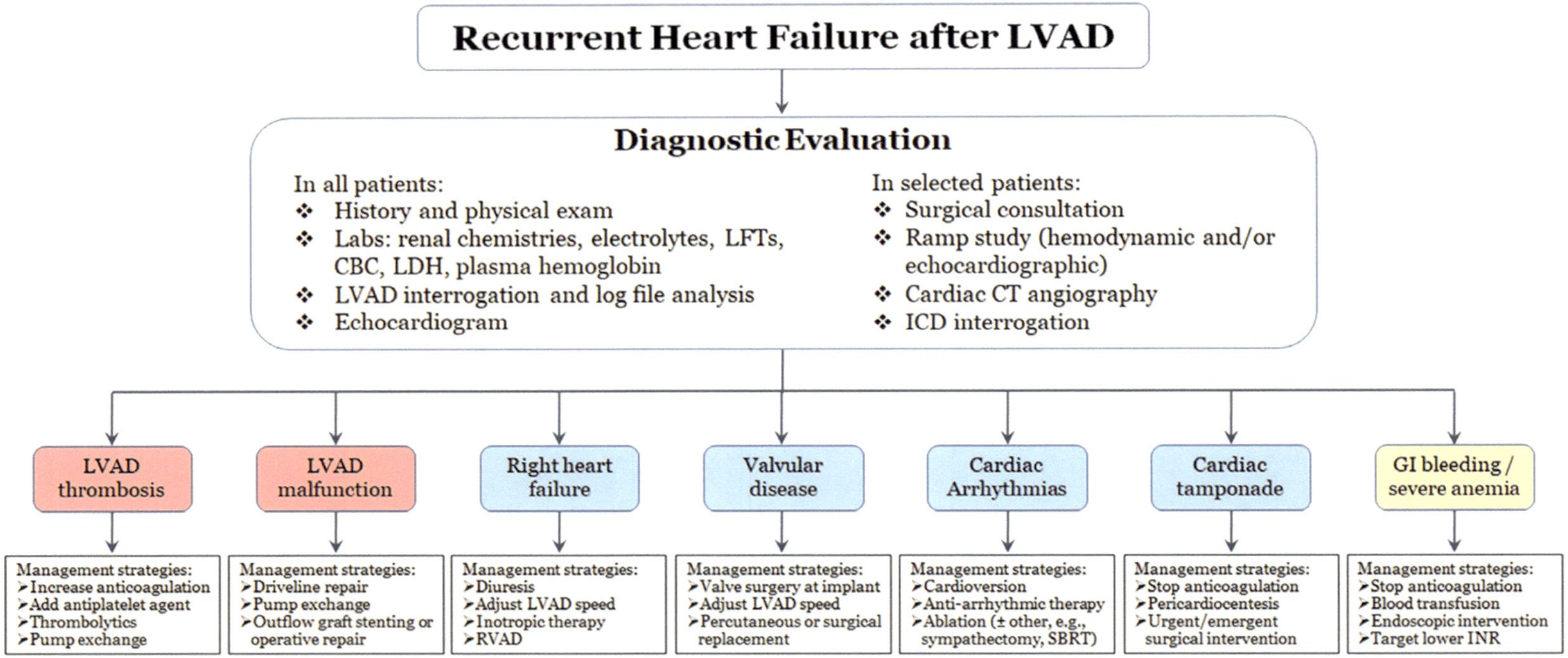

Figure 9.
Algorithm for the assessment and management of recurrent heart failure (HF) in the LVAD patient. Depending on the severity of the underlying lesion, patients may be hemodynamically stable or unstable at initial evaluation. In the unstable patient, a more targeted diagnostic evaluation should be performed to rapidly identify the cause of HF. LFT = liver function testing; CBC = complete blood count; LDH = lactate dehydrogenase; CT = computed tomography; ICD = implantable cardioverter defibrillator; SBRT = stereotactic body radiation therapy. LVAD-specific causes in red; intrinsic cardiac causes in blue; non-cardiac causes in yellow.

an RVAD after the initial operation. Concomitant RVAD implant was associated with >2-fold lower mortality vs. RVAD implant after completion of LVAD surgery [88]. In the IMACS registry, RVAD use was associated with substantially lower survival. Further, within the RVAD group, there was progressively worse survival with longer times between LVAD and RVAD surgery (1-year survival: LVAD only 82.9%; RVAD at time of LVAD implant, 58.5%; RVAD ≤14 days after LVAD, 51.6%; RVAD 15–30 days after LVAD, 32.4%) [30]. A major limitation of these studies is a lack of propensity matching and the inability to fully control for baseline differences, identifying an urgent area for future research.

3.1.2 Late right heart failure

There is almost no substantive data guiding management of late right HF. First, it is important to identify the cause of right HF (**Figure 2**). LVAD speed should be optimized and arrhythmias managed as indicated [89]. Importantly, the only manifestation of ventricular tachyarrhythmias in an LVAD patient may be HF. Pulmonary hypertension usually improves with offloading of the LV, but could worsen in the setting of MR. However, most cases of late right HF are likely due to intrinsic RV dysfunction in the myopathic heart.

As with early right HF, the cornerstone of therapy is diuresis. However, this is often insufficient and many patients require initiation of inotropic therapy. In patients developing late right HF in the STS-INTERMACS database, 33–50% required inotropic support [45]. Unfortunately, inotrope use portends a very poor prognosis with substantially elevated mortality even beyond those with late right HF that do not require inotropes [33, 45]. The need for extended inotrope use also increases the risk of infection due to chronic indwelling intravenous catheter placement, and may be associated with poorer functional status and QOL, though data are lacking. As no pumps are approved for hospital discharge, RVAD support is virtually never employed in late right HF, being used in <0.2% of those in the STS-INTERMACS database [45].

3.2 Management of Valvular Disease

Valve surgery at the time of LVAD implant is common and uniformly increases morbidity relative to LVAD surgery alone. Mortality data with valve surgery at the time of LVAD are mixed. In the HMII trials, 21.9% underwent valve surgery with modestly increased mortality (1-year survival: 69% vs. 75%, p = 0.004) [90]. In the ADVANCE trial, 19.6% had concomitant valve surgery, and though the absolute difference in survival was the same as with HMII, the result was not significant (79% vs. 85%, p = 0.33) [91]. In the MOMENTUM 3 CAP registry, 21.8% had valve surgery with equivalent survival at 2-years (81.7% vs. 80.8%, p = 0.6) [92]. Registry data show a similar prevalence of valve surgery at LVAD implant (IMACS, 12.1%; [30] EUROMACS, 19.3% [93]). When those having valve surgery in EUROMACS were propensity matched to LVAD patients not undergoing valve surgery, 1-year survival was the same (67.9% vs. 66.4%, p = 0.25) [93].

Notably, early right HF was actually higher with concurrent valve surgery in the HMII [90], ADVANCE [91], and HM 3 trials [92], while the propensity matched cohort in EUROMACS had equivalent rates of RVAD use [93]. Late right HF was not different in the HMII or ADVANCE trials but was increased with concurrent valve surgery in the MOMENTUM 3 CAP registry.

3.2.1 Aortic valve disease

Hemodynamically significant AI can be addressed via 3 methods (reviewed in detail elsewhere) [94]: (1) complete closure (oversewing) of the AV; (2) AV repair (e.g., central closure via Park's stitch [95]); or (3) AV replacement (AVR). Closure successfully eliminates AI, but acute LVAD malfunction may be rapidly fatal as this method leaves no native cardiac output. AV repair closes the central orifice of the AV while still allowing blood flow through the lateral commissures. This prevents blood stasis and thrombosis in the aortic root, and durably limits AI [94]. Of note, if AVR is pursued, mechanical valves are not recommended due to decreased valve opening and blood flow that could increase the chance of thrombosis.

Outcomes data distinguishing the best approach are extremely limited. Among those with concurrent AV and continuous flow LVAD surgery between 2006 and 2012 in INTERMACS, survival was lower with AV closure than either AV repair or AVR, suggesting that preservation of AV opening is beneficial [96]. More recent data from IMACS showed reduced survival with concurrent procedures, with AV repair having numerically better survival than AVR [70]. However, data were compared to no AV surgery, leaving unclear if the difference between repair and AVR was significant. In both studies, CPB time and LOS were longer with AV procedures.

Though mortality may be increased, residual confounding is possible due to the lack of prospective, randomized data. Whether AV procedures are of benefit in a subpopulation of LVAD patients remains unclear. Among concomitant AV procedures in IMACS, ~50% were performed in those with mild AI [70]. Interestingly, when this analysis was limited to those with moderate or severe AI, survival was the same between AV repair, AVR and those not receiving AV surgery. This suggests that the benefit may be restricted to those with more severe disease.

Finally, as noted, AI will develop and/or progress in the majority of LVAD patients (**Figure 8B**). Despite this, data on the optimal approach to these patients is markedly limited. Post-LVAD AI has been managed with (1) open AVR; (2) percutaneous closure of the aortic valve with an occlusion device (e.g., those used for septal defects); or (3) percutaneous AVR (TAVR). Percutaneous methods have increased over the last decade but no large-scale studies have been performed to study different approaches. In a meta-analysis of 15 case series (only 29 patients), percutaneous treatments were durable and showed no difference in mortality between occlusion or TAVR [97]. A study using the Nationwide Readmission Database found no difference in mortality between surgical AVR and TAVR but showed substantially lower morbidity with TAVR [98]. Given the prevalence of post-LVAD AI, this is an urgent area for future research.

3.2.2 Mitral valve disease

Intraoperative management of moderate or severe MR remains controversial. Among those with moderate or severe MR in INTERMACS, only 5.3% underwent MV surgery (95.8% repair, 4.2% replacement) at the time of LVAD [99]. MR severity 3-months after LVAD was equivalent in both groups (moderate/severe MR in 20% with MV procedure, 25% with LVAD alone, $p = 0.2$). Importantly, there was no survival benefit between: (1) those with moderate/severe MR undergoing LVAD and MV surgery vs. LVAD alone; (2) those with baseline moderate vs. severe MR; nor (3) those with baseline no/mild MR vs. moderate/severe. A trend ($p = 0.09$) towards benefit of concurrent MR surgery 2-years after LVAD was noted in DT patients. MV surgery was associated with longer LOS and CPB time, but fewer rehospitalizations. The incidence of right HF was the same and 6-minute walk distance was not different with or without concurrent MV surgery [99].

These data suggest there is little benefit to correcting MR at the time of LVAD and risk predictors have not been established to identify subgroups who might derive benefit. However, in INTERMACS, the presence of moderate or severe MR at least 3-months after LVAD implant was associated with a nearly 2-fold increased risk of right HF and a trend towards lower survival [75]. Data are lacking to guide management in LVAD patients with significant residual MR.

3.2.3 Tricuspid valve disease

Surgical treatment of moderate or severe TR at the time of LVAD is similarly controversial. Among those with moderate/severe TR in INTERMACS, 16.5% underwent TV surgery (>95% repair) at the time of LVAD [100]. TV surgery was associated with slightly lower survival (hazard ratio 1.13, p = 0.04) and significantly higher rates of stroke, bleeding and arrhythmia. Concurrent TV surgery did not impact patient-reported QOL [100]. In a propensity matched cohort from EUROMACS, TV surgery had no impact on survival, readmission, or right HF after LVAD [101]. Further, at 1-year, the prevalence of moderate or severe TR was similar between those with TV surgery or LVAD alone [101]. Other large single center studies have confirmed a high failure rate (~30–40%) of TV surgery in LVAD patients [102, 103]. Notably, the rate of concurrent TV surgery has declined in the last decade, possibly in response to the mounting evidence for a lack of benefit. Whether subgroups that do benefit can be identified remains to be determined.

3.3 Management of LVAD device malfunction

While failure of any part of the LVAD can be life threatening, the majority of issues with external components are readily remedied without harm [79]. By contrast, LVAD thrombosis almost always requires therapy (**Figure 9**). Pump or driveline failure triggering LVAD exchange occurred in 0.6% of HMII recipients in an early INTERMACS analysis [104]. Driveline malfunction (more common with the HMII than HVAD) rarely requires urgent intervention. Major driveline issues occurred in ~2.2% of >13,000 HMII patients, and of those only 20% required urgent surgical intervention (driveline repair, pump exchange, OHT) [105]. There are as yet no data on the incidence and outcomes of driveline issues with the HM3.

Lastly, LVAD cannula problems should also be considered in the differential diagnosis of recurrent HF. Although rare, malalignment of the inflow cannula may require surgical correction. Outflow cannula obstruction is predominantly caused by external compression of the outflow graft or stenosis of the aortic anastomosis [83]. While surgical correction is an option, the safety and long-term durability of outflow graft stenting has recently been confirmed and can be performed with very low morbidity [83].

4. Conclusions

Recurrent HF is a very common complication after LVAD implant and portends a poor prognosis with increased morbidity and mortality. The causes are varied and identifying the correct etiology is critically important to proper management (**Figure 9**).

Given the highly specialized nature of many of these etiologies, it is recommended that HF in the LVAD patient be managed in an active LVAD center. A wealth of evidence exists defining the incidence and prevalence of LVAD-associated HF. However, only limited data are available to guide therapies.

In our opinion, future research to reduce morbidity associated with recurrent HF should focus on 3 major areas. (1) Preemptive strategies to prevent right HF: for instance, pre-LVAD temporary MCS usage has increased with time in the STS-INTERMACS database [8], but whether it will impact post-VAD outcomes remains to be determined. (2) Perioperative improvements and standardization of surgical methods: for instance, a meta-analysis of LVAD implant via lateral thoracotomy suggests a significantly lower incidence of post-LVAD right HF, an approach being tested in the ongoing SWIFT trial [106]. And, finally, (3) prospective assessment to identify treatment strategies that provide significant benefit for patients with recurrent HF. These could be pharmacologic strategies, or possibly development of durable RV support. Regardless, the breathtaking pace of LVAD technological development will no doubt continue to benefit patients with advanced HF.

Conflict of interest

None

Author details

Tamas Alexy[1] and Michael A. Burke[2]*

1 Division of Cardiology, University of Minnesota, Minneapolis, USA

2 Cardiology Division, Emory University School of Medicine, Atlanta, USA

*Address all correspondence to: michael.burke@emory.edu

References

[1] Tsao CW, Aday AW, Almarzooq ZI, Alonso A, Beaton AZ, Bittencourt MS, et al. Heart disease and stroke Statistics-2022 update: A report from the American Heart Association. Circulation. 2022;**145**(8):e153-e639

[2] Bragazzi NL, Zhong W, Shu J, Abu Much A, Lotan D, Grupper A, et al. Burden of heart failure and underlying causes in 195 countries and territories from 1990 to 2017. European Journal of Preventive Cardiology. 2021;**28**(15):1682-1690

[3] Miller LW, Guglin M. Patient selection for ventricular assist devices: A moving target. Journal of the American College of Cardiology. 2013;**61**(12):1209-1221

[4] Kalogeropoulos AP, Samman-Tahhan A, Hedley JS, McCue AA, Bjork JB, Markham DW, et al. Progression to stage D heart failure among outpatients with stage C heart failure and reduced ejection fraction. JACC: Heart Failure. 2017;**5**(7):528-537

[5] Mancini D, Colombo PC. Left ventricular assist devices: A rapidly evolving alternative to transplant. Journal of the American College of Cardiology. 2015;**65**(23):2542-2555

[6] Organ Procurement and Transplantation Network. 2022. Available from: https://optn.transplant.hrsa.gov/data/view-data-reports/national-data/#. [Accessed: May 27, 2022]

[7] Mehra MR, Uriel N, Naka Y, Cleveland JC Jr, Yuzefpolskaya M, Salerno CT, et al. A fully magnetically levitated left ventricular assist device - final report. The New England Journal of Medicine. 2019;**380**(17):1618-1627

[8] Shah P, Yuzefpolskaya M, Hickey GW, Breathett K, Wever-Pinzon O, Ton VK, et al. Twelfth interagency registry for mechanically assisted circulatory support report: Readmissions after left ventricular assist device. The Annals of Thoracic Surgery. 2022;**113**(3):722-737

[9] Mehra MR, Cleveland JC Jr, Uriel N, Cowger JA, Hall S, Horstmanshof D, et al. Primary results of long-term outcomes in the MOMENTUM 3 pivotal trial and continued access protocol study phase: A study of 2200 HeartMate 3 left ventricular assist device implants. European Journal of Heart Failure. 2021;**23**(8):1392-1400

[10] Burke MA, Givertz MM. Assessment and management of heart failure after left ventricular assist device implantation. Circulation. 2014;**129**(10):1161-1166

[11] Ali HR, Kiernan MS, Choudhary G, Levine DJ, Sodha NR, Ehsan A, et al. Right ventricular failure post-implantation of left ventricular assist device: Prevalence, pathophysiology, and predictors. ASAIO Journal. 2020;**66**(6):610-619

[12] Rose EA, Gelijns AC, Moskowitz AJ, Heitjan DF, Stevenson LW, Dembitsky W, et al. Long-term use of a left ventricular assist device for end-stage heart failure. The New England Journal of Medicine. 2001;**345**(20):1435-1443

[13] Lietz K, Long JW, Kfoury AG, Slaughter MS, Silver MA, Milano CA, et al. Outcomes of left ventricular assist device implantation as destination therapy in the post-REMATCH era: Implications for patient selection. Circulation. 2007;**116**(5):497-505

[14] Slaughter MS, Rogers JG, Milano CA, Russell SD, Conte JV, Feldman D, et al. Advanced heart failure treated with continuous-flow left ventricular assist device. The New England Journal of Medicine. 2009;**361**(23):2241-2251

[15] Kirklin JK, Naftel DC, Kormos RL, Stevenson LW, Pagani FD, Miller MA, et al. Second INTERMACS annual report: More than 1,000 primary left ventricular assist device implants. The Journal of Heart and Lung Transplantation. 2010;**29**(1):1-10

[16] Molina EJ, Shah P, Kiernan MS, Cornwell WK 3rd, Copeland H, Takeda K, et al. The Society of Thoracic Surgeons Intermacs 2020 annual report. The Annals of Thoracic Surgery. 2021;**111**(3):778-792

[17] Clerkin KJ, Salako O, Fried JA, Griffin JM, Raikhelkar J, Jain R, et al. Impact of temporary percutaneous mechanical circulatory support before transplantation in the 2018 heart allocation system. JACC: Heart Failure. 2022;**10**(1):12-23

[18] Kormos RL, Antonides CFJ, Goldstein DJ, Cowger JA, Starling RC, Kirklin JK, et al. Updated definitions of adverse events for trials and registries of mechanical circulatory support: A consensus statement of the mechanical circulatory support academic research consortium. The Journal of Heart and Lung Transplantation. 2020;**39**(8):735-750

[19] STS Intermacs Database. 2022. Available from: https://www.uab.edu/medicine/intermacs/intermacs-documents. [Accessed: June 3, 2022]

[20] Konstam MA, Kiernan MS, Bernstein D, Bozkurt B, Jacob M, Kapur NK, et al. Evaluation and Management of Right-Sided Heart Failure: A scientific statement from the American Heart Association. Circulation. 2018;**137**(20):e578-e622

[21] Brown SB, Raina A, Katz D, Szerlip M, Wiegers SE, Forfia PR. Longitudinal shortening accounts for the majority of right ventricular contraction and improves after pulmonary vasodilator therapy in normal subjects and patients with pulmonary arterial hypertension. Chest. 2011;**140**(1):27-33

[22] Iglesias-Garriz I, Olalla-Gomez C, Garrote C, Lopez-Benito M, Martin J, Alonso D, et al. Contribution of right ventricular dysfunction to heart failure mortality: A meta-analysis. Reviews in Cardiovascular Medicine. 2012;**13**(2-3):e62-e69

[23] Morgan JA, Paone G, Nemeh HW, Murthy R, Williams CT, Lanfear DE, et al. Impact of continuous-flow left ventricular assist device support on right ventricular function. The Journal of Heart and Lung Transplantation. 2013;**32**(4):398-403

[24] Kiernan MS, Grandin EW, Brinkley M Jr, Kapur NK, Pham DT, Ruthazer R, et al. Early right ventricular assist device use in patients undergoing continuous-flow left ventricular assist device implantation: Incidence and risk factors from the interagency registry for mechanically assisted circulatory support. Circulation. Heart Failure. 2017;**10**:e003863

[25] Lampert BC, Teuteberg JJ. Right ventricular failure after left ventricular assist devices. The Journal of Heart and Lung Transplantation. 2015;**34**(9):1123-1130

[26] Rich JD. Right ventricular failure in patients with left ventricular assist devices. Cardiology Clinics. 2012;**30**(2):291-302

[27] Kormos RL, Teuteberg JJ, Pagani FD, Russell SD, John R, Miller LW, et al. Right ventricular failure in patients with the HeartMate II continuous-flow left ventricular assist device: Incidence, risk factors, and effect on outcomes. The Journal of Thoracic and Cardiovascular Surgery. 2010;**139**(5):1316-1324

[28] Aaronson KD, Slaughter MS, Miller LW, McGee EC, Cotts WG, Acker MA, et al. Use of an intrapericardial, continuous-flow, centrifugal pump in patients awaiting heart transplantation. Circulation. 2012;**125**(25):3191-3200

[29] de By T, Schoenrath F, Veen KM, Mohacsi P, Stein J, Alkhamees KMM, et al. The European registry for patients with mechanical circulatory support of the European Association for Cardio-Thoracic Surgery: Third report. European Journal of Cardio-Thoracic Surgery. 2022;**62**(1):ezac032

[30] Goldstein DJ, Meyns B, Xie R, Cowger J, Pettit S, Nakatani T, et al. Third annual report from the ISHLT mechanically assisted circulatory support registry: A comparison of centrifugal and axial continuous-flow left ventricular assist devices. The Journal of Heart and Lung Transplantation. 2019;**38**(4):352-363

[31] Rich JD, Gosev I, Patel CB, Joseph S, Katz JN, Eckman PM, et al. The incidence, risk factors, and outcomes associated with late right-sided heart failure in patients supported with an axial-flow left ventricular assist device. The Journal of Heart and Lung Transplantation. 2017;**36**(1):50-58

[32] Bellavia D, Iacovoni A, Scardulla C, Moja L, Pilato M, Kushwaha SS, et al. Prediction of right ventricular failure after ventricular assist device implant: Systematic review and meta-analysis of observational studies. European Journal of Heart Failure. 2017;**19**(7):926-946

[33] Kapelios CJ, Lund LH, Wever-Pinzon O, Selzman CH, Myers SL, Cantor RS, et al. Right heart failure following left ventricular device implantation: Natural history, risk factors, and outcomes: An analysis of the STS INTERMACS database. Circulation. Heart Failure. 2022;**15**:e008706

[34] Soliman OII, Akin S, Muslem R, Boersma E, Manintveld OC, Krabatsch T, et al. Derivation and validation of a novel right-sided heart failure model after implantation of continuous flow left ventricular assist devices: The EUROMACS (European registry for patients with mechanical circulatory support) right-sided heart failure risk score. Circulation. 2018;**137**(9):891-906

[35] Warren OJ, Smith AJ, Alexiou C, Rogers PL, Jawad N, Vincent C, et al. The inflammatory response to cardiopulmonary bypass: Part 1--mechanisms of pathogenesis. Journal of Cardiothoracic and Vascular Anesthesia. 2009;**23**(2):223-231

[36] Warren OJ, Watret al, de Wit KL, Alexiou C, Vincent C, Darzi AW, et al. The inflammatory response to cardiopulmonary bypass: Part 2--anti-inflammatory therapeutic strategies. Journal of Cardiothoracic and Vascular Anesthesia. 2009;**23**(3):384-393

[37] Estrada VH, Franco DL, Moreno AA, Gambasica JA, Nunez CC. Postoperative right ventricular failure in cardiac surgery. Cardiology Research. 2016;7(6):185-195

[38] Boyle AJ, Ascheim DD, Russo MJ, Kormos RL, John R, Naka Y, et al. Clinical outcomes for continuous-flow left ventricular assist device patients stratified by pre-operative

INTERMACS classification. The Journal of Heart and Lung Transplantation. 2011;**30**(4):402-407

[39] Anselmi A, Abbate A, Girola F, Nasso G, Biondi-Zoccai GG, Possati G, et al. Myocardial ischemia, stunning, inflammation, and apoptosis during cardiac surgery: A review of evidence. European Journal of Cardio-Thoracic Surgery. 2004;**25**(3):304-311

[40] Raina A, Vaidya A, Gertz ZM, Susan C, Forfia PR. Marked changes in right ventricular contractile pattern after cardiothoracic surgery: Implications for post-surgical assessment of right ventricular function. The Journal of Heart and Lung Transplantation. 2013;**32**(8):777-783

[41] Unsworth B, Casula RP, Yadav H, Baruah R, Hughes AD, Mayet J, et al. Contrasting effect of different cardiothoracic operations on echocardiographic right ventricular long axis velocities, and implications for interpretation of post-operative values. International Journal of Cardiology. 2013;**165**(1):151-160

[42] Argenziano M, Choudhri AF, Moazami N, Rose EA, Smith CR, Levin HR, et al. Randomized, double-blind trial of inhaled nitric oxide in LVAD recipients with pulmonary hypertension. The Annals of Thoracic Surgery. 1998;**65**(2):340-345

[43] Varma PK, Srimurugan B, Jose RL, Krishna N, Valooran GJ, Jayant A. Perioperative right ventricular function and dysfunction in adult cardiac surgery-focused review (part 2-management of right ventricular failure). Indian Journal of Thoracic and Cardiovascular Surgery. 2022;**38**(2):157-166

[44] Brescia AA, Watt TMF, Pagani FD, Cascino TM, Zhang M, McCullough JS, et al. Assessment of mortality among durable left ventricular assist device recipients ineligible for clinical trials. JAMA Network Open. 2021;**4**(1):e2032865

[45] Rame JE, Pagani FD, Kiernan MS, Oliveira GH, Birati EY, Atluri P, et al. Evolution of late right heart failure with left ventricular assist devices and association with outcomes. Journal of the American College of Cardiology. 2021;**78**(23):2294-2308

[46] Miller LW, Pagani FD, Russell SD, John R, Boyle AJ, Aaronson KD, et al. Use of a continuous-flow device in patients awaiting heart transplantation. The New England Journal of Medicine. 2007;**357**(9):885-896

[47] Park SJ, Milano CA, Tatooles AJ, Rogers JG, Adamson RM, Steidley DE, et al. Outcomes in advanced heart failure patients with left ventricular assist devices for destination therapy. Circulation. Heart Failure. 2012;**5**(2):241-248

[48] Strueber M, Larbalestier R, Jansz P, Zimpfer D, Fiane AE, Tsui S, et al. Results of the post-market registry to evaluate the HeartWare left ventricular assist system (ReVOLVE). The Journal of Heart and Lung Transplantation. 2014;**33**(5):486-491

[49] Mehra MR, Naka Y, Uriel N, Goldstein DJ, Cleveland JC Jr, Colombo PC, et al. A fully magnetically levitated circulatory pump for advanced heart failure. The New England Journal of Medicine. 2017;**376**(5):440-450

[50] Agrawal S, Garg L, Shah M, Agarwal M, Patel B, Singh A, et al. Thirty-day readmissions after left ventricular assist device implantation in the United States: Insights from the Nationwide readmissions

database. Circulation. Heart Failure. 2018;**11**(3):e004628

[51] Kapelios CJ, Charitos C, Kaldara E, Malliaras K, Nana E, Pantsios C, et al. Late-onset right ventricular dysfunction after mechanical support by a continuous-flow left ventricular assist device. The Journal of Heart and Lung Transplantation. 2015;**34**(12):1604-1610

[52] Teuteberg JJ, Cleveland JC Jr, Cowger J, Higgins RS, Goldstein DJ, Keebler M, et al. The Society of Thoracic Surgeons Intermacs 2019 annual report: The changing landscape of devices and indications. The Annals of Thoracic Surgery. 2020;**109**(3):649-660

[53] Starling RC, Estep JD, Horstmanshof DA, Milano CA, Stehlik J, Shah KB, et al. Risk assessment and comparative effectiveness of left ventricular assist device and medical Management in Ambulatory Heart Failure Patients: The ROADMAP study 2-year results. JACC: Heart Failure. 2017;**5**(7):518-527

[54] Takeda K, Naka Y, Yang JA, Uriel N, Colombo PC, Jorde UP, et al. Outcome of unplanned right ventricular assist device support for severe right heart failure after implantable left ventricular assist device insertion. The Journal of Heart and Lung Transplantation. 2014;**33**(2):141-148

[55] Reid G, Mork C, Gahl B, Appenzeller-Herzog C, von Segesser LK, Eckstein F, et al. Outcome of right ventricular assist device implantation following left ventricular assist device implantation: Systematic review and meta-analysis. Perfusion. 2021 [Online ahead of print]

[56] Vierecke J, Gahl B, de By T, Antretter H, Beyersdorf F, Caliskan K, et al. Results of primary biventricular support: An analysis of data from the EUROMACS registry. European Journal of Cardio-Thoracic Surgery. 2019;**56**(6):1037-1045

[57] Takeda K, Takayama H, Colombo PC, Jorde UP, Yuzefpolskaya M, Fukuhara S, et al. Late right heart failure during support with continuous-flow left ventricular assist devices adversely affects post-transplant outcome. The Journal of Heart and Lung Transplantation. 2015;**34**(5):667-674

[58] Taghavi S, Jayarajan SN, Komaroff E, Mangi AA. Right ventricular assist device results in worse post-transplant survival. The Journal of Heart and Lung Transplantation. 2016;**35**(2):236-241

[59] Immohr MB, Boeken U, Mueller F, Prashovikj E, Morshuis M, Bottger C, et al. Complications of left ventricular assist devices causing high urgency status on waiting list: Impact on outcome after heart transplantation. ESC Heart Failure. 2021;**8**(2):1253-1262

[60] Khush KK, Hsich E, Potena L, Cherikh WS, Chambers DC, Harhay MO, et al. The international thoracic organ transplant registry of the International Society for Heart and Lung Transplantation: Thirty-eighth adult heart transplantation report - 2021; focus on recipient characteristics. The Journal of Heart and Lung Transplantation. 2021;**40**(10):1035-1049

[61] Truby LK, Farr MA, Garan AR, Givens R, Restaino SW, Latif F, et al. Impact of bridge to transplantation with continuous-flow left ventricular assist devices on Posttransplantation mortality. Circulation. 2019;**140**(6):459-469

[62] King PM, Raymer DS, Shuster J, Crain M, Bhatia A, Hartupee J, et al. Right heart failure while on left ventricular assist device support is associated with primary graft

dysfunction. ASAIO Journal. 2020;**66**(10):1137-1141

[63] Cowger JA, Naka Y, Aaronson KD, Horstmanshof D, Gulati S, Rinde-Hoffman D, et al. Quality of life and functional capacity outcomes in the MOMENTUM 3 trial at 6 months: A call for new metrics for left ventricular assist device patients. The Journal of Heart and Lung Transplantation. 2018;**37**(1):15-24

[64] Grandin EW, Troutman GS, Gulati AA, Zamani P, Mazurek JA, Atluri P, et al. A modified grading system for early right heart failure matches functional outcomes and survival after left ventricular assist devices. ASAIO Journal. 2021;**67**(2):185-191

[65] Kiernan MS, Sundareswaran KS, Pham DT, Kapur NK, Pereira NL, Strueber M, et al. Preoperative determinants of quality of life and functional capacity response to left ventricular assist device therapy. Journal of Cardiac Failure. 2016;**22**(10):797-805

[66] Guglin M, Verma S. Right side of heart failure. Heart Failure Reviews. 2012;**17**(3):511-527

[67] Frankfurter C, Molinero M, Vishram-Nielsen JKK, Foroutan F, Mak S, Rao V, et al. Predicting the risk of right ventricular failure in patients undergoing left ventricular assist device implantation: A systematic review. Circulation. Heart Failure. 2020;**13**(10):e006994

[68] Feldman D, Pamboukian SV, Teuteberg JJ, Birks E, Lietz K, Moore SA, et al. The 2013 International Society for Heart and Lung Transplantation guidelines for mechanical circulatory support: Executive summary. The Journal of Heart and Lung Transplantation. 2013;**32**(2):157-187

[69] Truby LK, Garan AR, Givens RC, Wayda B, Takeda K, Yuzefpolskaya M, et al. Aortic insufficiency during contemporary left ventricular assist device support: Analysis of the INTERMACS registry. JACC: Heart Failure. 2018;**6**(11):951-960

[70] Veenis JF, Yalcin YC, Brugts JJ, Constantinescu AA, Manintveld OC, Bekkers JA, et al. Survival following a concomitant aortic valve procedure during left ventricular assist device surgery: An ISHLT mechanically assisted circulatory support (IMACS) registry analysis. European Journal of Heart Failure. 2020;**22**(10):1878-1887

[71] Rajagopal K, Daneshmand MA, Patel CB, Ganapathi AM, Schechter MA, Rogers JG, et al. Natural history and clinical effect of aortic valve regurgitation after left ventricular assist device implantation. The Journal of Thoracic and Cardiovascular Surgery. 2013;**145**(5):1373-1379

[72] Cowger J, Pagani FD, Haft JW, Romano MA, Aaronson KD, Kolias TJ. The development of aortic insufficiency in left ventricular assist device-supported patients. Circulation. Heart Failure. 2010;**3**(6):668-674

[73] Gasparovic H, Kopjar T, Saeed D, Cikes M, Svetina L, Petricevic M, et al. De novo aortic regurgitation after continuous-flow left ventricular assist device implantation. The Annals of Thoracic Surgery. 2017;**104**(2):704-711

[74] Kanwar MK, Rajagopal K, Itoh A, Silvestry SC, Uriel N, Cleveland JC Jr, et al. Impact of left ventricular assist device implantation on mitral regurgitation: An analysis from the MOMENTUM 3 trial. The Journal of Heart and Lung Transplantation. 2020;**39**(6):529-537

[75] Jain R, Truby LK, Topkara VK. Residual mitral regurgitation in patients with left ventricular assist device support - an INTERMACS analysis. The Journal of Heart and Lung Transplantation. 2022 [Online ahead of print]

[76] Veen KM, Mokhles MM, Soliman O, de By T, Mohacsi P, Schoenrath F, et al. Clinical impact and 'natural' course of uncorrected tricuspid regurgitation after implantation of a left ventricular assist device: An analysis of the European registry for patients with mechanical circulatory support (EUROMACS). European Journal of Cardio-Thoracic Surgery. 2021;**59**(1):207-216

[77] Nakanishi K, Homma S, Han J, Takayama H, Colombo PC, Yuzefpolskaya M, et al. Prevalence, predictors, and prognostic value of residual tricuspid regurgitation in patients with left ventricular assist device. Journal of the American Heart Association. 2018;**7**(13):e008813

[78] Mehra MR, Salerno C, Naka Y, Uriel N, Cleveland JC, Horstmanshof D, et al. A tale of the twist in the outflow graft: An analysis from the MOMENTUM 3 trial. The Journal of Heart and Lung Transplantation. 2018;**37**(11):1281-1284

[79] Kormos RL, McCall M, Althouse A, Lagazzi L, Schaub R, Kormos MA, et al. Left ventricular assist device malfunctions: It is more than just the pump. Circulation. 2017;**136**(18):1714-1725

[80] Zimpfer D, Gustafsson F, Potapov E, Pya Y, Schmitto J, Berchtold-Herz M, et al. Two-year outcome after implantation of a full magnetically levitated left ventricular assist device: Results from the ELEVATE registry. European Heart Journal. 2020;**41**(39):3801-3809

[81] Chivukula VK, Beckman JA, Prisco AR, Dardas T, Lin S, Smith JW, et al. Left ventricular assist device inflow cannula angle and thrombosis risk. Circulation. Heart Failure. 2018;**11**(4):e004325

[82] Imamura T, Nguyen A, Chung B, Rodgers D, Sarswat N, Kim G, et al. Association of Inflow Cannula Position with left ventricular unloading and clinical outcomes in patients with HeartMate II left ventricular assist device. ASAIO Journal. 2019;**65**(4):331-335

[83] Agrawal A, Alexy T, Kamioka N, Shafi T, Stowe J, Morris AA, et al. Outflow graft obstruction after left ventricular assist device implantation: A retrospective, single-Centre case series. ESC Heart Failure. 2021;**8**(3):2349-2353

[84] Uriel N, Burkhoff D, Rich JD, Drakos SG, Teuteberg JJ, Imamura T, et al. Impact of hemodynamic ramp test-guided HVAD speed and medication adjustments on clinical outcomes. Circulation. Heart Failure. 2019;**12**(4):e006067

[85] Cogswell R, John R, Shaffer A. Right ventricular failure after left ventricular assist device. Cardiology Clinics. 2020;**38**(2):219-225

[86] McCullough M, Caraballo C, Ravindra NG, Miller PE, Mezzacappa C, Levin A, et al. Neurohormonal blockade and clinical outcomes in patients with heart failure supported by left ventricular assist devices. JAMA Cardiology. 2020;**5**(2):175-182

[87] Brinkley DM Jr, Wang L, Yu C, Grandin EW, Kiernan MS. Impact of renin-angiotensin-aldosterone system inhibition on morbidity and mortality during long-term continuous-flow left ventricular assist device support:

An IMACS report. The Journal of Heart and Lung Transplantation. 2021;**40**(12):1605-1613

[88] Kumar S, Derbala MH, Nguyen DT, Ferrall J, Cefalu M, Rivas-Lasarte M, et al. A multi-institutional retrospective analysis on impact of RV acute mechanical support timing after LVAD implantation on 1-year mortality and predictors of RV acute mechanical support weaning. The Journal of Heart and Lung Transplantation. 2022;**41**(2):244-254

[89] Kadado AJ, Akar JG, Hummel JP. Arrhythmias after left ventricular assist device implantation: Incidence and management. Trends in Cardiovascular Medicine. 2018;**28**(1):41-50

[90] John R, Naka Y, Park SJ, Sai-Sudhakar C, Salerno C, Sundareswaran KS, et al. Impact of concurrent surgical valve procedures in patients receiving continuous-flow devices. The Journal of Thoracic and Cardiovascular Surgery. 2014;**147**(2):581-589

[91] Milano C, Pagani FD, Slaughter MS, Pham DT, Hathaway DR, Jacoski MV, et al. Clinical outcomes after implantation of a centrifugal flow left ventricular assist device and concurrent cardiac valve procedures. Circulation. 2014;**130**(11 Suppl. 1):S3-S11

[92] John R, Kanwar MK, Cleveland JC Jr, Uriel N, Naka Y, Salerno C, et al. Concurrent valvular procedures during left ventricular assist device implantation and outcomes: A comprehensive analysis of the Multicenter study of MagLev Technology in Patients Undergoing Mechanical Circulatory Support Therapy with HeartMate 3 trial portfolio. The Journal of Thoracic and Cardiovascular Surgery. 2022 [Online ahead of print]

[93] Loforte A, de By T, Gliozzi G, Schonrath F, Mariani C, Netuka I, et al. Impact of concomitant cardiac valvular surgery during implantation of continuous-flow left ventricular assist devices: A European registry for patients with mechanical circulatory support (EUROMACS) analysis. Artificial Organs. 2022;**46**(5):813-826

[94] Goodwin ML, Bobba CM, Mokadam NA, Whitson BA, Essandoh M, Hasan A, et al. Continuous-flow left ventricular assist devices and the aortic valve: Interactions, issues, and surgical therapy. Current Heart Failure Reports. 2020;**17**(4):97-105

[95] Park SJ, Liao KK, Segurola R, Madhu KP, Miller LW. Management of aortic insufficiency in patients with left ventricular assist devices: A simple coaptation stitch method (Park's stitch). The Journal of Thoracic and Cardiovascular Surgery. 2004;**127**(1):264-266

[96] Robertson JO, Naftel DC, Myers SL, Prasad S, Mertz GD, Itoh A, et al. Concomitant aortic valve procedures in patients undergoing implantation of continuous-flow left ventricular assist devices: An INTERMACS database analysis. The Journal of Heart and Lung Transplantation. 2015;**34**(6):797-805

[97] Phan K, Haswell JM, Xu J, Assem Y, Mick SL, Kapadia SR, et al. Percutaneous Transcatheter interventions for aortic insufficiency in continuous-flow left ventricular assist device patients: A systematic review and Meta-analysis. ASAIO Journal. 2017;**63**(2):117-122

[98] Zaidi SH, Minhas AMK, Sagheer S, ManeshGangwani K, Dani SS, Goel SS, et al. Clinical outcomes of Transcatheter aortic valve replacement (TAVR) vs. surgical aortic valve replacement (SAVR)

in patients with durable left ventricular assist device (LVAD). Current Problems in Cardiology. 2022;**47**:101313

[99] Robertson JO, Naftel DC, Myers SL, Tedford RJ, Joseph SM, Kirklin JK, et al. Concomitant mitral valve procedures in patients undergoing implantation of continuous-flow left ventricular assist devices: An INTERMACS database analysis. The Journal of Heart and Lung Transplantation. 2018;**37**(1):79-88

[100] Mullan C, Caraballo C, Ravindra NG, Miller PE, Mori M, McCullough M, et al. Clinical impact of concomitant tricuspid valve procedures during left ventricular assist device implantation. The Journal of Heart and Lung Transplantation. 2020;**39**(9):926-933

[101] Veen KM, Caliskan K, de By T, Mokhles MM, Soliman OI, Mohacsi P, et al. Outcomes after tricuspid valve surgery concomitant with left ventricular assist device implantation in the EUROMACS registry: A propensity score matched analysis. European Journal of Cardio-Thoracic Surgery. 2019;**56**(6):1081-1089

[102] Barac YD, Nicoara A, Bishawi M, Schroder JN, Daneshmand MA, Hashmi NK, et al. Durability and efficacy of tricuspid valve repair in patients undergoing left ventricular assist device implantation. JACC: Heart Failure. 2020;**8**(2):141-150

[103] Fujino T, Imamura T, Nitta D, Kim G, Smith B, Kalantari S, et al. Effect of concomitant tricuspid valve surgery with left ventricular assist device implantation. The Annals of Thoracic Surgery. 2020;**110**(3):918-924

[104] Holman WL, Naftel DC, Eckert CE, Kormos RL, Goldstein DJ, Kirklin JK. Durability of left ventricular assist devices: Interagency registry for mechanically assisted circulatory support (INTERMACS) 2006 to 2011. The Journal of Thoracic and Cardiovascular Surgery. 2013;**146**(2):437-441

[105] Kalavrouziotis D, Tong MZ, Starling RC, Massiello A, Soltesz E, Smedira NG, et al. Percutaneous lead dysfunction in the HeartMate II left ventricular assist device. The Annals of Thoracic Surgery. 2014;**97**(4):1373-1378

[106] Ribeiro RVP, Lee J, Elbatarny M, Friedrich JO, Singh S, Yau T, et al. Left ventricular assist device implantation via lateral thoracotomy: A systematic review and meta-analysis. The Journal of Heart and Lung Transplantation. 2022 [Online ahead of print]

Chapter 6

Aortic Insufficiency in LVAD Patients

Vi Vu and Karen May-Newman

Abstract

Aortic insufficiency (AI) is a common complication that increases morbidity and mortality in patients with left ventricular assist devices (LVAD). Significant AI during LVAD support creates a substantial regurgitant flow loop, negatively affecting cardiac recovery and exposing blood to longer residence time and higher shear stress. The mechanism of AI development and progression is linked to a lack of aortic valve opening, which alters the valvular tissue mechanics. Pre-existing AI also worsens following LVAD implantation, interfering with the pump benefits. This chapter will evaluate AI development with LVAD support compared with naturally occurring AI and present the features, mechanisms, and links to clinical treatment options.

Keywords: aortic valve, insufficiency, LVAD, flow, aortic insufficiency (AI)

1. Introduction

Moderate-severe aortic insufficiency (AI) develops in more than 25% of left ventricular assist device (LVAD) recipients and reduces survival and freedom from other complications. Improvements in LVAD design have not addressed this problem, which continues to threaten the benefits of mechanical circulatory support. AI can develop de novo or progress from pre-existing AI conditions [1–7] and is associated primarily with rotary LVADs, also called continuous flow pumps. AI occurs when the mitral valve does not close completely during diastolic filling (**Figure 1**). The large pressure difference across the valve produces retrograde flow from the aorta to the LV. During LVAD support, the retrograde flow passes through the LVAD and into the ascending aorta, and a portion joins the regurgitant flow to repeat the cycle, exposing the blood to more shear. Significant AI diminishes cardiac output, negatively affects myocardial recovery and induces end-organ hypoperfusion [1]. Previous studies have linked a lack of aortic valve (AV) opening to the development of AI. Alterations in AV biomechanics during LVAD support can increase the activation of valvular interstitial cells, which transform into myofibroblasts that increase fibrosis preferentially at the ventricular face of the leaflets and fusion at the commissures. The subsequent contraction of fibrotic tissue and the fragmentation of elastin reduces coaptation, eventually resulting in AI. Assessment of AI in LVAD patients must be adapted from standard guidelines to determine when treatment is needed.

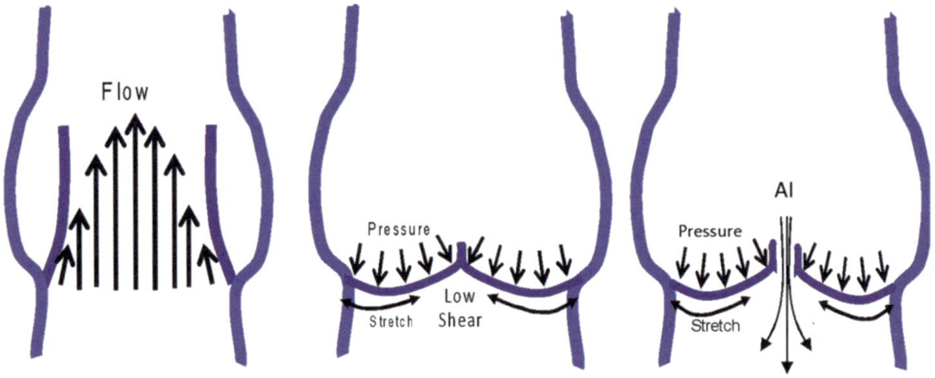

Figure 1.
Schematic of aortic insufficiency (AI), when the aortic valve leaks under high pressures, reducing forward flow.

2. Clinical complications of aortic insufficiency during LVAD support

Aortic insufficiency occurs when the AV does not close completely, thus inducing a backward flow from the aorta to the left ventricle (LV). As severe AI progresses, usually over many years, valve repair or replacement is needed to resolve the problem. Naturally occurring affects 0.5% of the general population and 2% of those over 75 years and is responsible for only 4% of all deaths from AV disease [8]. However, for LVAD patients, AI is a significant complication that occurs in more than 25% of recipients and has persisted despite improvements in design, surgical placement, and control.

The most recent INTERMACS report noted an average LVAD support duration of 1.7 years and a comparable survival rate in axial and centrifugal continuous-flow LVAD [9]. For axial and centrifugal LVAD designs, the leading causes of death are similar, including neurologic dysfunction, multisystem organ failure, infection, and stroke (ischemic or hemorrhagic) [9]. Moreover, the risk of readmission due to severe adverse events increases as patients stay longer in LVAD support [9]. Some recurrent adverse events with rates noted at 1 year post-implant are shown in **Figure 2** [9–12].

As LVADs are implanted for longer support durations, complications related to tissue remodeling or other adaptations to the altered physiology introduced by the LVAD arise. AI is one of those, appearing within a few months of LVAD support and worsening over time [6, 13, 14]. Reports of AI were not common for the early pulsatile LVADs but have risen with the implantation of rotary LVADs of axial and centrifugal designs. Many of these clinical studies are single-center with relatively few patients. Still, a consistent picture has emerged that ~15% of patients develop AI within three months of LVAD support, and the fraction increases to ~25% at 12 months and over 30% after 3 years (**Figure 3**) [1, 6, 12–16].

Rotary LVADs include axial designs, like the HeartMateII, which operate at high speeds and have a linear flow path through the housing. Centrifugal LVAD designs such as the HeartMate3 direct blood along a radial path, from the center towards the side, and operate at lower speeds which is gentler for the blood. Some LVADs have added speed modulation to introduce pulsatility to the flow, improving the washout to prevent thrombi from forming inside of the LVAD. These innovations have reduced hemolysis and thromboembolic complications but have not substantially reduced the occurrence of AI.

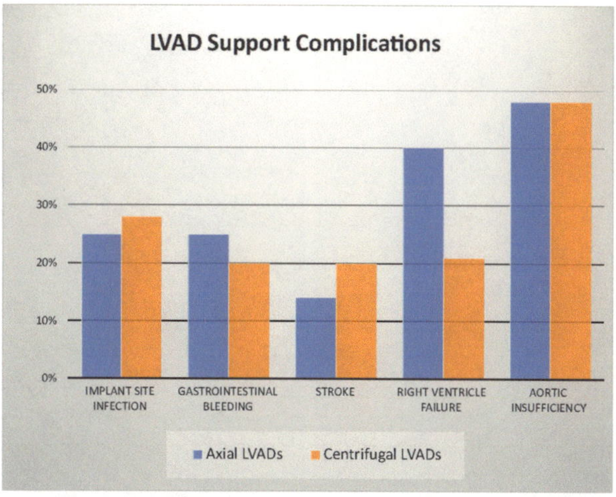

Figure 2.
Complications of left ventricular assist device (LVAD) support [9–12].

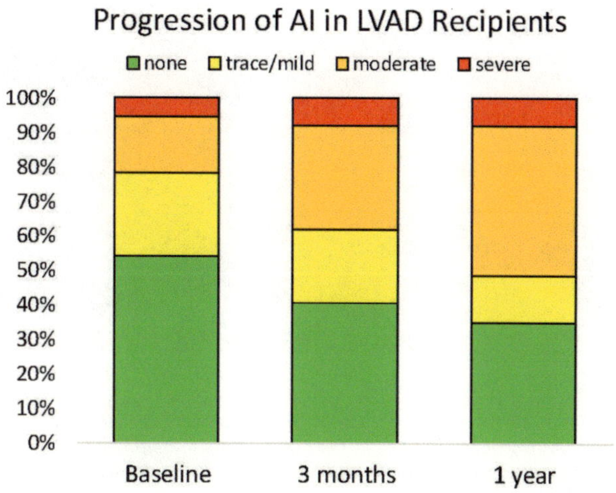

Figure 3.
Graphical illustration of AI progression in LVAD patients shows a progress worsening within the first-year post-implant. Adapted from Imamura 2020 [16].

The progression of AI with LVAD support is well documented, but the underlying mechanisms remain unclear [17, 18]. Even mild AI that is unrepaired is associated with a higher incidence of AI progression to moderate/severe and worse NYHA functional class compared to trace or less AI patients in mid-term after LVAD implantation [19]. AI in LVAD recipients can occur de novo or progress from pre-existing AI conditions [1–3, 5–7]. De novo AI develops as early as three months post-implant, and freedom from significant AI decreases as LVAD support duration increases [12, 13, 15]. Long LVAD support duration and low ejection fraction have been identified as independent predictors of de novo AI development [2, 7].

When pre-existing AI is present, the severity tends to increase with time post-implant [1, 16]. LVAD support induced a larger regurgitant flow resulting in lower cardiac output, higher preload, and impacting HF status [18, 20, 21]. Worsening of

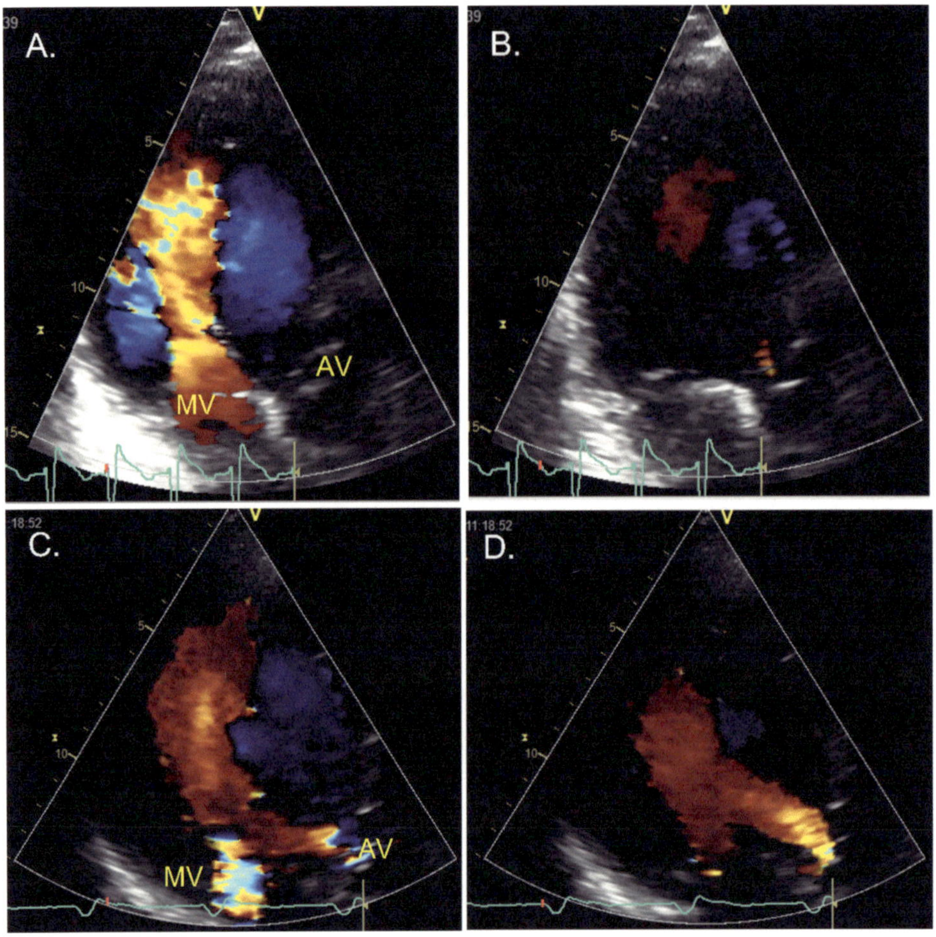

Figure 4.
Three-chambered echo view of LVAD patients with mild AI (top) and moderate/severe AI (bottom). A. Early diastolic filling through the mitral valve (MV). B. Mid diastole shows a small regurgitant jet through the aortic valve (AV). C-D. a large regurgitant jet appears in early diastole and merges with mitral inflow.

AI increases LVAD flow while systemic flow decreases, forming a regurgitant flow loop [21]. As shown in **Figure 4**, mild AI presents in mid-diastole but extends in magnitude and duration towards moderate/severe levels within a few months of LVAD support.

Moreover, LVAD patient with concurrent AI is associated with a higher readmission rate and adverse events, including mitral and tricuspid regurgitation, hemolysis, and worsening of right ventricle function [6, 20, 22]. Previous clinical studies have reported multiple factors associated with the worsening of pre-existing trivial AI in post-LVAD support. Patient-related factors included pre-existing valvular dysfunctions, old age, and abnormal cardiac function. Pre-existing valvular dysfunctions include uncorrected mild AI [23, 24], large aortic sinus diameters [6, 25], LVAD-related factors include reduction of AV opening area and duration, high LVAD speed, and types of LVAD [6, 25]. Previous studies have suggested that the higher rate of progressive AI with rotary LVAD support results from low pulsatility, which may induce a more significant regurgitant flow and a higher rate of valvular remodeling [22, 26–28].

3. Flow dynamics of aortic insufficiency during LVAD support

For the majority of rotary LVADs, the LVAD inlet is located at the LV apex, and the outlet anastomoses to the ascending aorta, bypassing the AV. Implantation of the LVAD immediately increases systemic blood flow and end-organ perfusion, providing an alternate pathway for blood to flow from the heart to the arterial system, as shown in **Figure 5**. LVAD support unloads the heart, decreasing the magnitude and pulsatility of LV pressure, which can fall below the level needed to open the AV fully during myocardial contraction. With sufficient contraction of the native heart, a fraction of the flow is ejected through the AV, and the heart and LVAD operate in parallel. In this condition, the AV does not open fully, exhibiting a reduced opening area and duration [29]. During periods of high LVAD support, the LV pressure is too small to open the AV, and blood flow occurs entirely through the LVAD, the heart, and the pump operating in series [30]. The AV is continuously closed for this condition and chronically exposed to high transvalvular pressure. For many patients, the level of LVAD support needed to relieve the HF symptoms results in complete and continuous closure of the AV, with all blood exiting the heart through the LVAD.

Adding a rotary LVAD to the native heart reduces the range of pressure and flow experienced in the cardiovascular system, diminishing pulsatility. The last decade of LVAD therapy has revealed several significant complications that worsen with reduced pulsatility, including thrombus formation, AV incompetence, and vascular smooth muscle response [17, 31]. The latter has been tied to arteriovenous malformations and gastrointestinal bleeding [17, 32]. Indices of pulsatility include pulse pressure, normalized flow range, and surplus hemodynamic energy [28, 30], which decrease as LVAD speed increases. When the AV ceases to open, the abnormal flow pattern creates a region of flow stasis adjacent to the AV, which creates a high risk for thromboembolism that could be embolized by a sudden strong contraction of the native heart [33].

Blood flow in the normal healthy heart is unsteady, 3-D and shows a range of different length scales [34]. A typical flow pattern in the LV has been described as consisting of a large diastolic vortex that channels the transit of incoming blood from the mitral valve towards the AV [35]. This vortex contributes to diastolic suction and minimizes kinetic energy losses and cardiac work [36]. The LV vortex has been shown to facilitate the blood mass coming into the normal LV during one beat washing out completely after a few beats [37], which prevents intraventricular blood stagnation [38].

In the LV of a diseased heart, progressive adverse remodeling leads to abnormal flow patterns that may impair pumping efficiency, and therefore affects blood transit within the ventricle. It is believed these abnormal intraventricular flow dynamics may contribute to the progression of certain diseases, leading to a final stage of HF or thrombus formation [39]. In addition, previous studies of flow transport through the heart have correlated dilated cardiomyopathy with increased vortex kinetic energy and decreased flow transport [40]. Models of this pathological condition have identified a high thrombus risk in DCM patients with large regions of blood flow with residence times greater than 2 s that also exhibit low kinetic energy [41]. When AI is present, retrograde flow mixing with the forward flow during diastole contributes to energy loss and increases residence time [41].

Thrombus formation and growth in several locations have been observed clinically, contributing to the high stroke rate in LVAD patients [42]. When AI develops in LVAD patients, the backward flow through the AV may improve pulsatility and flow stasis in

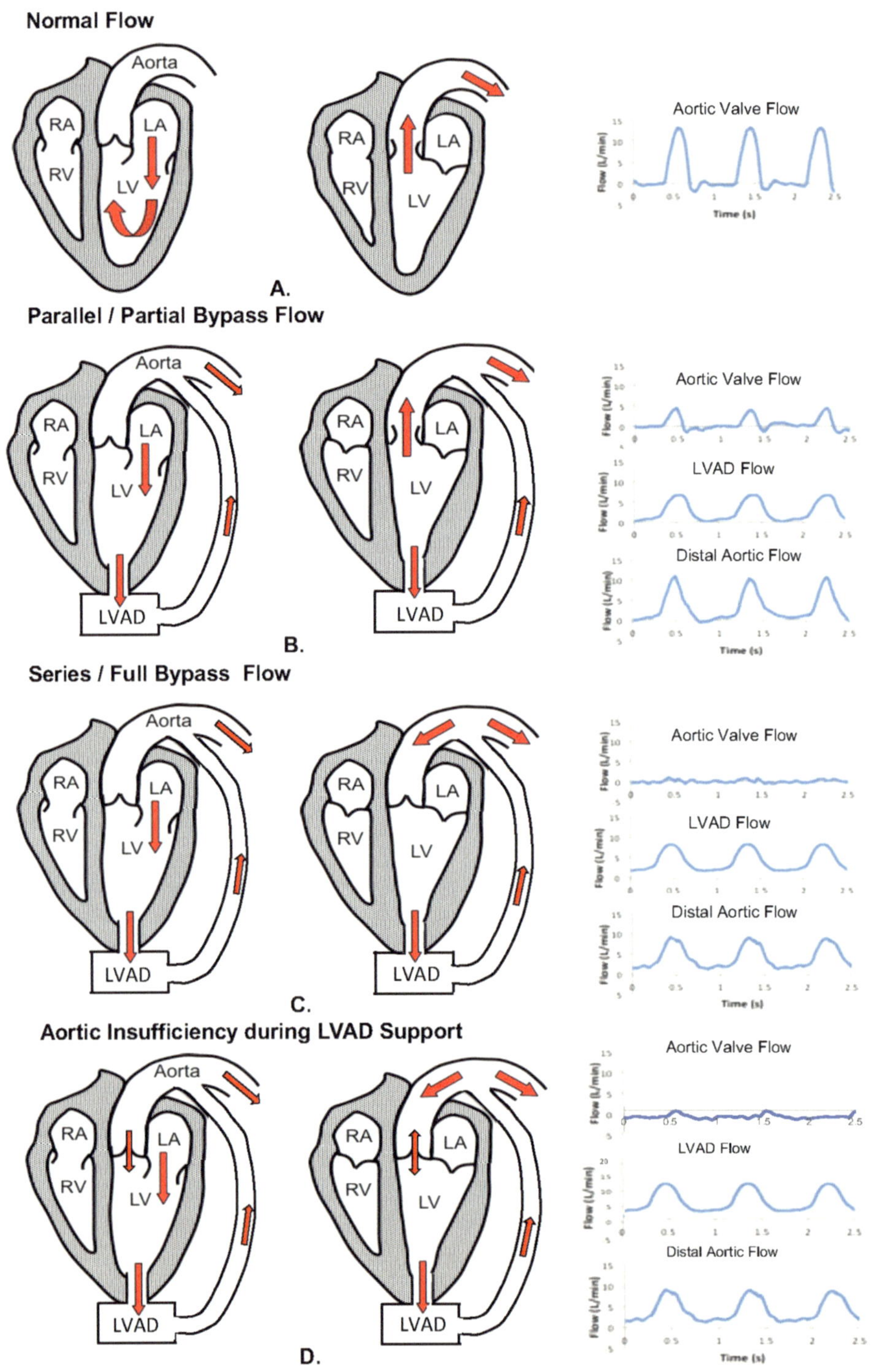

Figure 5.
Schematic of flow conditions. A. the normal flow path enters the left ventricle (LV) through the mitral valve and exits through the aortic valve and into the aorta. B. Low LVAD support works with the native heart to produce parallel flow through the LVAD and aortic valve. C. High LVAD support maintains continuous closure of the aortic valve during series flow. D. Aortic insufficiency produces retrograde flow through the aortic valve that can re-enter the LVAD in a regurgitant flow loop.

the aortic root, but over time results in reduced systemic flow. In particular, AI results in the formation of a regurgitant flow loop, in which blood from the LVAD flows retrograde through the AV, into the LV, and out through the LVAD again. This loop extends the amount and time-history of shear stress exposure to the blood, increasing hemolysis and thrombogenicity. The pump will also need to run at a higher speed to achieve the original cardiac output, which increases wear on the device. Hemostasis and thromboregulation are already compromised in LVAD patients, and AI adds to this liability.

During LVAD support, LV vortex formation is relatively unaffected, although vortex circulation and kinetic energy increase with LVAD speed, particularly in systole when all flow exits through the LVAD. When AI occurs, the regurgitant jet forms a vortex ring that normally dissipates in the mid-ventricle when no LVAD support is present but collides with the incoming mitral flow, as shown in **Figure 6**. When the LVAD is added, the regurgitant jet is drawn towards the LVAD inflow, impinging on the vortex ring generated by mitral inflow. The oppositely rotating vortices are partially annihilated, dissipating energy in the process. This flow pattern contributes to fluid stasis along the septal wall.

Recent device improvements include an "artificial pulse", based on a rapid LVAD speed change, that produces a small hemodynamic boost. While this artificial pulse provides substantial improvement in pulsatility, it is not synchronized with the native heartbeat and thus offers minimal improvement in the overall flow. The presence of speed modulation does not appear to impact the development of AI, which remains a significant complication of LVADs.

4. Aortic valve biomechanics during LVAD support

Human heart valves change their shapes and size during the cardiac cycle in response to their surrounding hemodynamics [43]. This mechanism helps facilitate the leaflet function and reduces the effect of flexural stress on the valve surface [43]. An average heart valve opens and closes more than three billion times in a lifetime and experiences various stress and strain types (e.g., tensile, compressive, stretching, and bending) [43]. The AV is a thin tissue structure with three leaflets attached to the aortic root wall in a u-shaped pattern in a roughly symmetric arrangement. Each leaflet forms a pocket with the corresponding sinus, which plays a vital role in the fluid mechanics of opening and closing [44]. During diastolic filling, the valve is closed, and the leaflets stretch in opposition to the high transvalvular pressure [17]. When the AV opens during systole, the leaflets relax as blood flows over the ventricular surface and into the aorta. Some of the flow is captured as vortices that form behind the valve leaflets, ensuring smooth closure. The unidirectional laminar blood flow produces shear stress of up to 80 dynes/cm^2 on the ventricular endothelial surface [45]. In contrast, the aortic surface has a small magnitude oscillatory flow in the range of ±10 dyn/cm^2 shear stress [46].

During LVAD support, the pressure difference across the AV remains high for a longer fraction of the cardiac cycle, producing a decrease in flow that corresponds to a reduction in valve opening. The valve opening area decreases with LVAD support, with more of the valve commissures coapted over the entire cardiac cycle. LVAD support also reduces the duration of AV opening, which increases the time that the leaflet tissue experiences maximum pressure loading. Simultaneously, the shear across the ventricular surface of the valve leaflet is reduced and eventually eliminated when the AV remains closed.

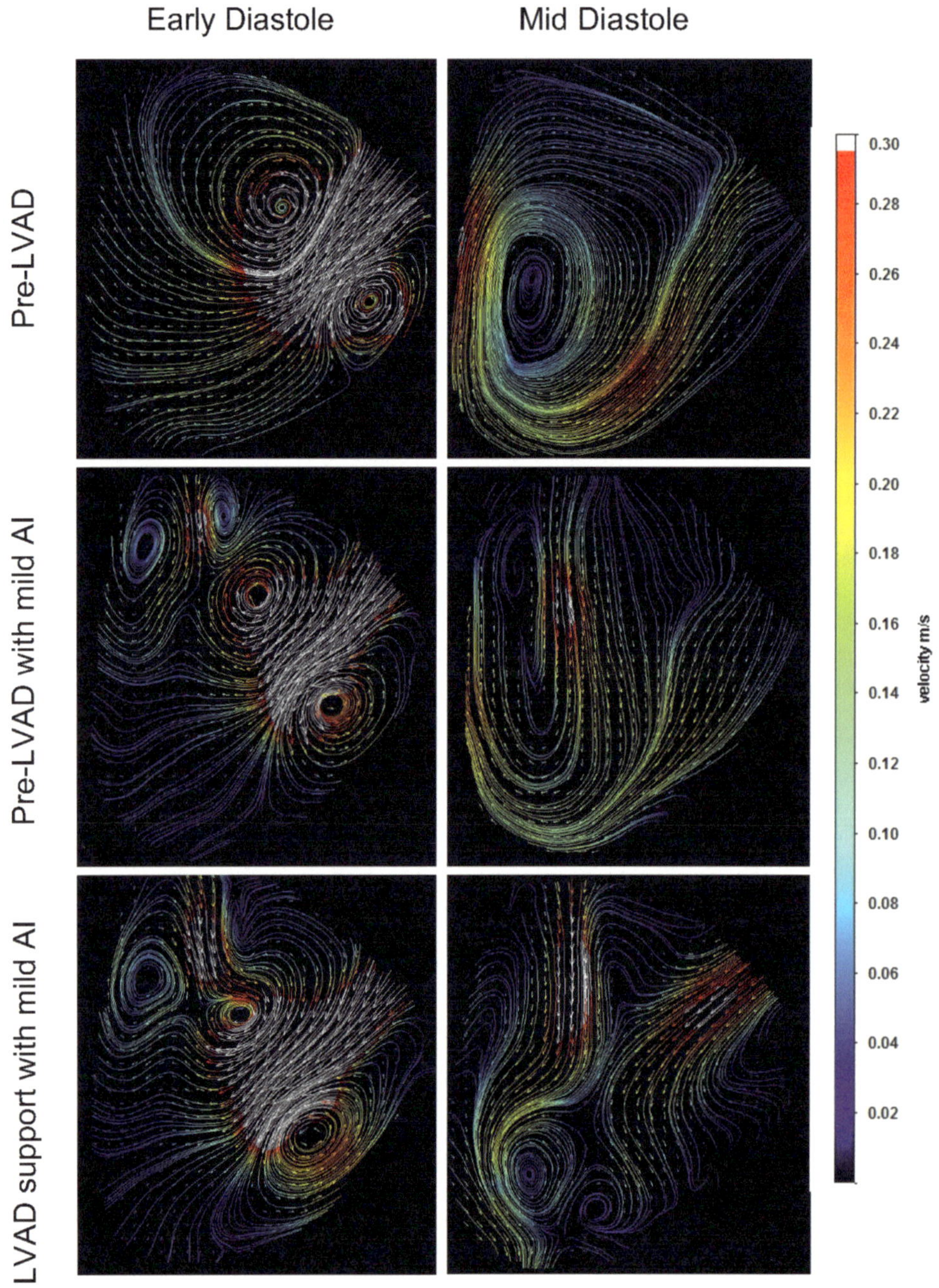

Figure 6.
Flow field images during early and mid-diastole illustrate the vortex ring generated by the regurgitant jet that collides with the mitral valve inflow.

At the level of the valve tissue and cells, the impact of LVAD hemodynamics produces a sudden change in the mechanical signals that can initiate a sequence of remodeling that results in AI. Measurements of valve tissue stretch during LVAD support show that the aortic leaflets are stiffer in the circumferential direction and

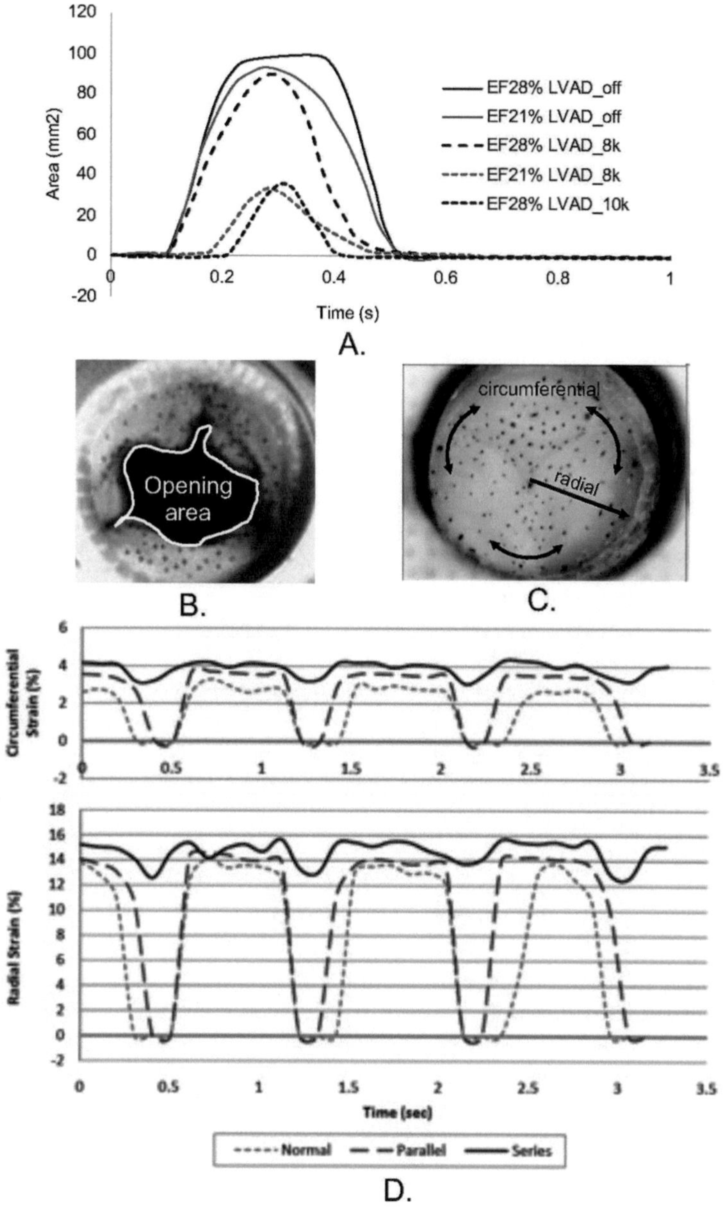

Figure 7.
A. Aortic valve opening area and duration with different cardiac function and LVAD support, B. Aortic valve opening area, C. Surface marker movement was used to measure stretch in the circumferential (hoop) and radial directions D. Stretch is highest for series flow when the aortic valve remains closed.

more compliant in the radial direction. This behavior corresponds to the alignment of collagen fibers with the circumferential direction, termed the anisotropy of the tissue. The peak stretch increases and extends for a longer duration as the normal flow pattern is compared to LVAD parallel and series conditions (**Figure 7**). Thus, the valve tissue experiences large and continuous tensile loading and significantly reduced ventricular shear during LVAD support.

5. Aortic valve commissural fusion during LVAD support

The AV leaflet tissue varies in thickness, being thicker at the free margin and annulus and thinner in the belly and coaptation areas. The leaflet tissue is composed of a layered structure of collagen, elastin, and proteoglycans. The textured fibrosa is a dense layer of circumferentially oriented collagen along the aortic face and bears most of the mechanical load [47]. The smooth ventricularis is an elastin layer adjacent to the ventricle, and the spongiosa is a central layer of loose connective tissue [47]. Naturally arising AV disease is preceded by tissue changes that occur over decades. Previous studies have shown that these are side-specific [48], manifesting as focal lesions that form preferentially from the aortic face, whereas the ventricular face is relatively disease-protected [49].

Post-transplant evaluation of LVAD-supported hearts has revealed the presence of extensive tissue remodeling of the AV, particularly commissural fusion, in 71–88% of LVAD patients [50, 51]. Aortic leaflet fusion creates adhesions between adjacent leaflets, preventing the complete opening of the valve [52, 53]. Increased fusion has been correlated with a longer duration of LVAD support [1, 6, 20] and with the development of AI [4, 51–53]. The aortic leaflets become more fibrotic and lose their elastic layer in the fusion areas, resulting in pathological remodeling, which progresses from the annulus towards the center of the valve (**Figure 8**). In contrast to naturally occurring AV disease, focal lesions arise from the ventricularis layer on the opposite side, as shown in **Figure 9** [17]. The hypothesis for this manifestation of valve dysregulation is that the high and continuous transvalvular pressure produces stretch and bending that is highest in the ventricular layer, activating a cellular process that results in extracellular matrix alterations. Fibrotic tissue often undergoes a consolidation and contraction stage, which preferentially affects the ventricular surface and may contribute to the improper coaptation that produces AI.

6. Valve mechanobiology during LVAD support

As explained previously, the addition of the LVAD to the heart results in a sudden increase in the pressure loading of the AV, in which tensile stress is increased, and shear is attenuated [54]. Each of these mechanical signals has been shown to play an important role in the progression of AV disease [43]. Evidence for the impact of LVAD-related increased tensile stretch and reduced shear stress on valve leaflets is found in extensive studies evaluating the role of mechanobiology in calcific AV

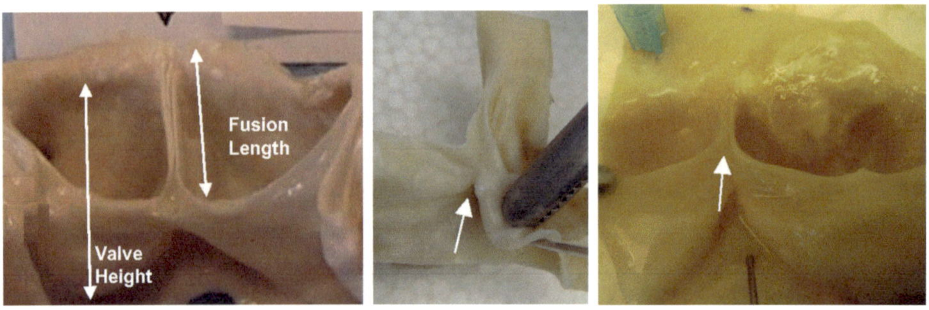

Figure 8.
Images of complete (left) and partial (center and right; location at the white arrow) commissural fusion of aortic valve leaflets following LVAD support.

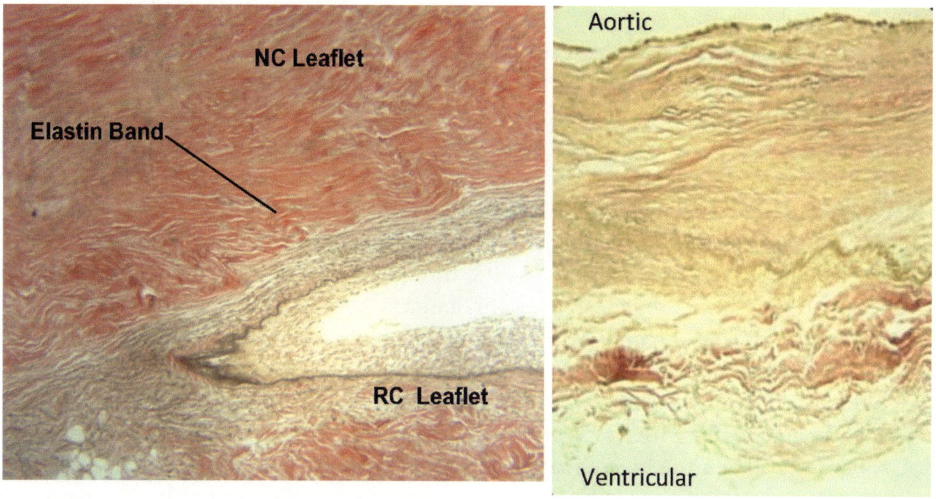

Figure 9.
Microscopic evaluation of aortic valve fusion from LVAD-supported hearts shows evidence of loss of the elastin band where the leaflets fuse together (left) and fibrosis arising from the ventricular face (right).

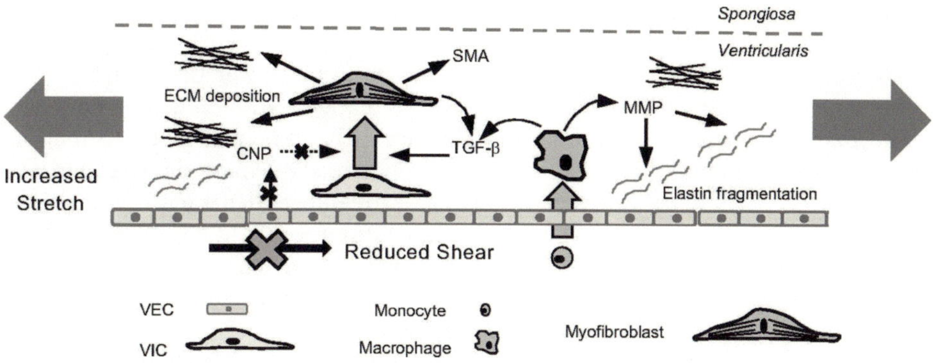

Figure 10.
LVAD support produces increased stretch and reduced shear in the ventricular layer of the aortic valve leaflet, which initiates a response resulting in ECM deposition and elastin fragmentation. The subsequent contraction of collagen in the ventricularis reduces leaflet coaptation, eventually resulting in AI.

disease and is illustrated in **Figure 10**. While this pathology manifests over a longer time and usually arises from the aortic surface of the leaflet, the same cell types are present in LVAD patients and respond to biochemical cues in the same way.

The cells responsible for valve tissue remodeling include the valvular endothelial cells (VECs), which reside in a single layer along the blood-contacting surfaces, and valvular interstitial cells (VICs), the more abundant cell type that resides throughout the tissue and is responsible for extracellular matrix maintenance [43]. VICs are usually quiescent and fibroblast-like but can be activated by abrupt changes in mechanical stress or when in a diseased state. VICs may translate between phenotypes to maintain homeostasis and can subsequently differentiate into other cell types, such as myofibroblasts, once activated [55]. Increased stretch provides a stimulus for VICs to increase collagen production and remodeling [56] by upregulating growth factors and integrins as cell-signaling mediators [57]. Stretch-activated VICs increase the production of collagen and remodeling enzymes, which can lead to fibrosis and calcification. As the disease progresses, the differentiation of VICs to myofibroblasts can be identified by increased α smooth muscle actin (α-SMA) expression. Myofibroblasts secrete ECM such as collagen and increase tension in the matrix fibers [58, 59] and are associated with the formation of ECM disarray and fibrosis [17, 30, 60]. Tissue macrophages synthesize enzymes associated with pathological remodeling, such as MMPs, that are not released by VICs. These enzymes degrade elastin, disrupt collagen organization [61, 62] and potentiate the pathological differentiation of VICs into myofibroblasts.

The pathological differentiation of VICs into myofibroblasts is promoted by large numbers of tissue macrophages in the ventricularis layer, which contributes to the overproduction of TGF-β. Side-specific shear also plays a key role in modulating the valve tissue. VECs on the aortic side of normal valves, which experience low shear, have reduced expression of many cytokines that are known inhibitors of fibrosis and calcification compared with VECs on the ventricular side, which normally experience high shear [59]. When the high shear is virtually eliminated, as occurs with LVAD support, the expression of C-type natriuretic peptide (CNP), a paracrine factor shown to inhibit VIC differentiation, is reduced [59]. The reduction in CNP coupled with a dramatic increase in TGF-β further accelerates the population of myofibroblasts [63].

7. Prevention and treatment of AI in LVAD patients

The goals for AI management are to treat the symptoms, lower long-term consequences, and improve patient outcomes [64]. Patients with mild-moderate AI and normal aortic root size, or asymptomatic severe AI and regular LV size/function are usually managed with vasodilators [65], although many debates the effectiveness in delaying AV repair or replacement [64, 66]. Meanwhile, patients with symptomatic severe AI, asymptomatic severe AI, and systolic dysfunction/LV dilation require surgical management [67, 68]. Mild-moderate AI is often corrected at the time of LVAD implantation, especially in long-term supported patients, or in those with larger body sizes and large aortic root diameters (>3.3 cm) [6, 23, 69].

Surgical treatment is selected based on the candidate's underlying pathology, LVAD support duration, and INTERMACS classification to allow the possibility of LV recovery by maintaining the native AV structure and function (**Figure 11**) [6, 69–71]. Without any repair procedure, pre-existing mild AI is three times more likely to progress to moderate-severe AI [23]. Other complications worsen in the long term, including right ventricle dysfunction, mitral and tricuspid regurgitations [24].

7.1 Partial closure central park stitch/modified park stitch

The Park Stitch includes a single, pledgeted 4–0 Prolene suture placed at the central portion of the AV leaflets [70]. It is effective when the original valvular tissue is sufficiently thick and has enough tensile strength to hold the sutures. Alternatively, the modified Park stitch, consisting of stitches securing pledgets with individual commissural at the AV center, is recommended when the valve leaflets are relatively thin [72]. The recipients are monitored carefully during LVAD speed regulation and ramp testing to avoid stitch rupture from sudden AV opening [18]. These techniques have debatable durability: at 4–6 months post-implant, approximately 20% moderate-worse AI recurrence rate occurred in some centers [69, 73], while others reported a much lower rate (0 to 7%) [6, 72].

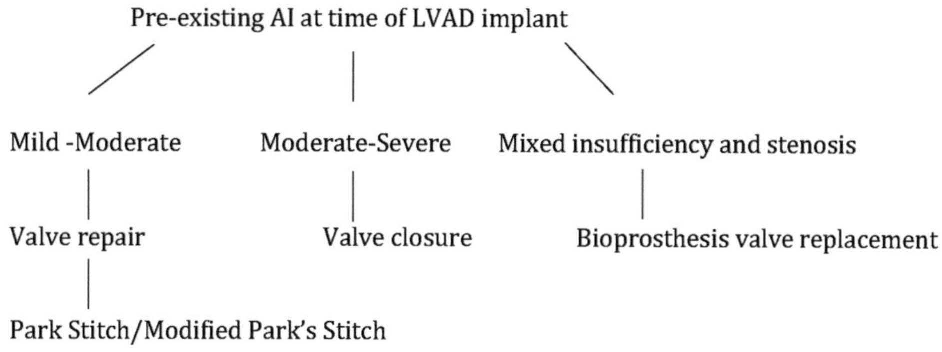

Figure 11.
Summary of the current treatment guidelines for pre-existing AI at the time of LVAD implant [6, 69–71].

7.2 Complete valve closure

Complete AV closure is recommended for patients with degenerative AV (leaflet prolapse or mal-coaptation) [18]. This procedure is performed by suturing felt strips to the leaflets or using a patch to cover the valve annulus directly. In the presence of a bioprosthesis, the valve is removed, and a pericardial patch is used to close the outflow tract [71, 74]. This procedure is durable with no AV deterioration or recurrent AI but induces a potential risk of thrombosis and restricts the possibility of myocardial recovery [18, 69, 71].

7.3 AV replacement

In patients with mixed stenosis or calcific pathology and insufficient AV, the valve can be replaced with a bioprosthesis. While allowing the possibility of AV opening, myocardial recovery, and pump removal, the limitations include a high risk of thrombosis, leaflet fusion, or stenosis [18, 21].

In post-LVAD patient management, AV structure and AI progression are monitored with routine echocardiography [75]. Intermittent AV opening was found to reduce the risk of AI development and improve LV systolic function and ejection fraction (especially in patients with preoperative short HF duration) [5, 6, 20, 22]. Optimization of pump speed (defined as the lowest possible LVAD support level to maintain adequate cardiac output and oxygen) is generally performed in case of mild AI to prevent worsening [6, 76]. If the patient's condition does not improve, surgical intervention will be performed. Approximately 5–10% of LVAD patients require AI-correction procedures after three or more years of LVAD support [6].

8. Conclusion

AI is a common complication affecting morbidity and mortality in LVAD patients. While the de novo AI development mechanism is unknown, it was linked to commissural fusion, lack of AV opening, and alteration of valvular tissue mechanics. Pre-existing AI also worsens in post-LVAD, interfering with the pump benefits.

Author details

Vi Vu* and Karen May-Newman
San Diego State University, San Diego, CA, USA

*Address all correspondence to: vtvu@sdsu.edu

References

[1] Cowger J, Pagani FD, Haft JW, Romano MA, Aaronson KD, Kolias TJ. The development of aortic insufficiency in left ventricular assist device-supported patients. Circulation. Heart Failure. 2010;**3**(6):668-674

[2] Aggarwal A, Raghuvir R, Eryazici P, Macaluso G, Sharma P, Blair C, et al. The development of aortic insufficiency in continuous-flow left ventricular assist device–supported patients. The Annals of Thoracic Surgery. 2013;**95**(2):493-498

[3] Bryant AS, Holman WL, Nanda NC, Vengala S, Blood MS, Pamboukian SV, et al. Native aortic valve insufficiency in patients with left ventricular assist devices. The Annals of Thoracic Surgery. 2006;**81**(2):e6-e8

[4] Samuels LE, Thomas MP, Holmes EC, Narula J, Fitzpatrick J, Wood D, et al. Insufficiency of the native aortic valve and left ventricular assist system inflow valve after support with an implantable left ventricular assist system: Signs, symptoms, and concerns. The Journal of Thoracic and Cardiovascular Surgery. 2001;**122**(2):380-381

[5] Pak SW, Uriel N, Takayama H, Cappleman S, Song R, Colombo PC, et al. Prevalence of de novo aortic insufficiency during long-term support with left ventricular assist devices. The Journal of Heart and Lung Transplantation. 2010;**29**(10):1172-1176

[6] Jorde UP, Uriel N, Nahumi N, Bejar D, Gonzalez-Costello J, Thomas SS, et al. Prevalence, significance, and Management of Aortic Insufficiency in continuous flow left ventricular assist device recipients. Circulation. Heart Failure. 2014;7(2):310-319

[7] Ben-ali W, Bouhout I, Lambert J, Bouchard D, Carrier M. Prevalence and impact of de novo aortic insufficiency during long-term support on a left ventricular assist device: A SYSTEMATIC review and META-analysis. Canadian Journal of Cardiology. 2017;**33**(10):S68-S69

[8] Coffey S, Cox B, Williams MJA. Lack of progress in valvular heart disease in the pre–transcatheter aortic valve replacement era: Increasing deaths and minimal change in mortality rate over the past three decades. American Heart Journal. 2014;**167**(4):562-567.e2

[9] Kormos RL, Cowger J, Pagani FD, Teuteberg JJ, Goldstein DJ, Jacobs JP, et al. The Society of Thoracic Surgeons Intermacs database annual report: Evolving indications, outcomes, and scientific partnerships. The Journal of Heart and Lung Transplantation. 2019;**38**(2):114-126

[10] Grant ADM, Smedira NG, Starling RC, Marwick TH. Independent and incremental role of quantitative right ventricular evaluation for the prediction of right ventricular failure after left ventricular assist device implantation. Journal of the American College of Cardiology. 2012;**60**(6):521-528

[11] Schlöglhofer T, Wittmann F, Paus R, Riebandt J, Schaefer AK, Angleitner P, et al. When nothing goes right: Risk factors and biomarkers of right heart failure after left ventricular assist device implantation. Life. 2022;**12**(3):459

[12] Malick A, Ning Y, Kurlansky PA, Melehy A, Yuzefpolskaya M, Colombo PC, et al. Development of De novo aortic insufficiency in patients with HeartMate 3.

The Annals of Thoracic Surgery. Aug 2022;**114**(2):450-456

[13] Truby LK, Garan AR, Givens RC, Wayda B, Takeda K, Yuzefpolskaya M, et al. Aortic insufficiency during contemporary left ventricular assist device support. JACC. Heart Failure. 2018;**6**(11):951-960

[14] Deo SV, Sharma V, Cho YH, Shah IK, Park SJ. De novo aortic insufficiency during long-term support on a left ventricular assist device: A Systematic review and Meta-analysis. ASAIO Journal. 2014;**60**(2):183-188

[15] Patil NP, Sabashnikov A, Mohite PN, Garcia D, Weymann A, Zych B, et al. De novo aortic regurgitation after continuous-flow left ventricular assist device implantation. The Annals of Thoracic Surgery. 2014;**98**(3):850-857

[16] Imamura T, Narang N, Kim G, Nitta D, Fujino T, Nguyen A, et al. Aortic insufficiency during HeartMate 3 left ventricular assist device support. Journal of Cardiac Failure. Oct 2020;**26**(10):863-869

[17] John R, Mantz K, Eckman P, Rose A, May-Newman K. Aortic valve pathophysiology during left ventricular assist device support. Journal of Heart and Lung Transplantation. Dec 2010;**29**(12):1321-1329

[18] Cowger J, Rao V, Massey T, Sun B, May-Newman K, Jorde U, et al. Comprehensive review and suggested strategies for the detection and management of aortic insufficiency in patients with a continuous-flow left ventricular assist device. Journal of Heart and Lung Transplantation. Feb 2015;**34**(2):149-157

[19] Tanaka Y, Nakajima T, Fischer I, Kotkar K, Moon M, Damiano R, et al. The Impact of Uncorrected Mild Aortic Insufficiency at the Time of Left Ventricular Assist Device Implantation. Toronto, Canada: AATS Annual Meeting; 2019

[20] Cowger JA, Aaronson KD, Romano MA, Haft J, Pagani FD. Consequences of aortic insufficiency during long-term axial continuous-flow left ventricular assist device support. The Journal of Heart and Lung Transplantation. 2014;**33**(12):1233-1240

[21] Garcia MAZ, Enriquez LA, Dembitsky W, May-Newman K. The effect of aortic valve incompetence on the hemodynamics of a continuous flow ventricular assist device in a mock circulation. ASAIO Journal. 2008;**54**(3):237-244

[22] Imamura T, Kinugawa K, Fujino T, Inaba T, Maki H, Hatano M, et al. Aortic insufficiency in patients with sustained left ventricular systolic dysfunction after axial flow assist device implantation. Circulation Journal. 2014;**79**(1):104-111

[23] Fukuhara S, Ikegami H, Polanco AR, Song JJ, Han J, Takeda K, et al. Concomitant repair for mild aortic insufficiency and continuous-flow left ventricular assist devices. European Journal of Cardio-Thoracic Surgery. 2017;**52**(6):1062-1068

[24] Tanaka Y, Nakajima T, Fischer I, Wan F, Kotkar K, Moon MR, et al. The impact of uncorrected mild aortic insufficiency at the time of left ventricular assist device implantation. The Journal of Thoracic and Cardiovascular Surgery. Dec 2020;**160**(6):1490-1500.e3

[25] Imamura T, Kinugawa K. Preoperative prediction of aortic

insufficiency during ventricular assist device treatment. International Heart Journal. 2016;**57**(1):3-10

[26] Gregory SD, Stevens MC, Wu E, Fraser JF, Timms D. In vitro evaluation of aortic insufficiency with a rotary left ventricular assist device. Artificial Organs. Sep 2013;**37**(9):802-809

[27] Stanfield JR, Selzman CH. In vitro Pulsatility analysis of axial-flow and centrifugal-flow left ventricular assist devices. Journal of Biomechanical Engineering. 2013;**135**(3):034505

[28] Soucy KG, Koenig SC, Giridharan GA, Sobieski MA, Slaughter MS. Defining pulsatility during continuous-flow ventricular assist device support. The Journal of Heart and Lung Transplantation. 2013;**32**(6):581-587

[29] Tolpen S, Janmaat J, Reider C, Kallel F, Farrar D, May-Newman K. Programmed speed reduction enables aortic valve opening and increased Pulsatility in the LVAD-assisted heart. ASAIO Journal. 2015;**61**(5):540-547

[30] Travis AR, Giridharan GA, Pantalos GM, Dowling RD, Prabhu SD, Slaughter MS, et al. Vascular pulsatility in patients with a pulsatile- or continuous-flow ventricular assist device. Journal of Thoracic and Cardiovascular Surgery. 2007;**133**(2):517-524

[31] May-Newman K, Wong YK, Adamson R, Hoagland P, Vu V, Dembitsky W. Thromboembolism is linked to intraventricular flow stasis in a patient supported with a left ventricle assist device. ASAIO Journal. 2013;**59**(4):452-455

[32] Lopilato AC, Doligalski CT, Caldeira C. Incidence and risk factor analysis for gastrointestinal bleeding and pump thrombosis in left ventricular assist device recipients: Hemostastic complications in LVAD recipients. Artificial Organs. 2015;**39**: 11, 939-944

[33] Mahr C, Chivukula VK, McGah P, Prisco AR, Beckman JA, Mokadam NA, et al. Intermittent aortic valve opening and risk of thrombosis in ventricular assist device patients. ASAIO Journal. 2017;**63**(4):425-432

[34] Hendabadi S, Bermejo J, Benito Y, Yotti R, Fernandez-Aviles F, del Alamo JC, et al. Topology of blood transport in the human left ventricle by novel processing of Doppler echocardiography. Annals of Biomedical Engineering. 2013;**41**:12, 2603-2616

[35] Martinez-Legazpi P, Bermejo J, Benito Y, Yotti R, Perez Del Villar C, Gonzalez-Mansilla A, et al. Contribution of the diastolic vortex ring to left ventricular filling. Journal of the American College of Cardiology. 2014;**64**(16):1711-1721

[36] Pedrizzetti G, Domenichini F. Nature optimizes the swirling flow in the human left ventricle. Physical Review Letters. 2005;**95**(10):1-4

[37] Watanabe H, Sugiura S, Hisada T. The looped heart does not save energy by maintaining the momentum of blood flowing in the ventricle. American Journal of Physiology Heart and Circulatory Physiology. 2008;**294**(5):H2191-H2196

[38] Hong GR, Pedrizzetti G, Tonti G, Li P, Wei Z, Kim JK, et al. Characterization and quantification of vortex flow in the human left ventricle by contrast echocardiography using vector particle image velocimetry. JACC Cardiovascular Imaging. 2008;**1**(6):705-717

[39] Carlha CJ, Bolger A. Advances in heart failure passing strange flow in the failing ventricle. Circulation Heart Failure. 2010;**3**:326-331

[40] Bermejo J, Benito Y, Alhama M, Yotti R, Martinez-Legazpi P, Del Villar CP, et al. Intraventricular vortex properties in nonischemic dilated cardiomyopathy. American Journal of Physiology Heart and Circulatory Physiology. 2014;**306**(5):H718-H729

[41] Rossini L, Braun OÖ, Brambatti M, Benito Y, Mizeracki A, Miramontes M, et al. Intraventricular flow patterns in patients treated with left ventricular assist devices. ASAIO Journal. 2021;**67**(1):74-83

[42] Kirklin JK, Naftel DC, Kormos RL, Pagani FD, Myers SL, Stevenson LW, et al. Interagency registry for mechanically assisted circulatory support (INTERMACS) analysis of pump thrombosis in the HeartMate II left ventricular assist device. Journal of Heart and Lung Transplantation. 2014;**33**(1):12-22

[43] Sacks MS, Yoganathan AP. Heart valve function: a biomechanical perspective. Philosophical Transactions of the Royal Society B: Biological Sciences. 2007;**362**(1484):1369-1391

[44] Beck A, Thubrikar MJ, Robicsek F. Stress analysis of the aortic valve with and without the sinuses of valsalva. The Journal of Heart Valve Disease. 2001;**10**(1):1-11

[45] Weston MW, LaBorde DV, Yoganathan a P. Estimation of the shear stress on the surface of an aortic valve leaflet. Annals of Biomedical Engineering. 1999;**27**(4):572-579

[46] Ge L, Sotiropoulos F. Direction and magnitude of blood flow shear stresses on the leaflets of aortic valves: Is there a link with valve calcification? Journal of Biomechanical Engineering. 2010;**132**(1):14505

[47] Thubrikar M. The Aortic Valve. Boca Raton, FL: CRC Press; 1989

[48] Sider KL, Blaser MC, Simmons CA. Animal models of calcific aortic valve disease. International Journal of Inflammation. 2011;**2011**:364310

[49] Yip CYY, Simmons C. a. the aortic valve microenvironment and its role in calcific aortic valve disease. Cardiovascular pathology: the Official Journal of the Society for Cardiovascular Pathology. 2011;**20**(3):177-182

[50] Mudd JO, Cuda JD, Halushka M, Soderlund KA, Conte JV, Russell SD. Fusion of aortic valve commissures in patients supported by a continuous axial flow left ventricular assist device. The Journal of Heart and Lung Transplantation. 2008;**27**(12):1269-1274

[51] May-Newman K, Mendoza A, Abulon DJK, Joshi M, Kunda A, Dembitsky W. Geometry and fusion of aortic valves from pulsatile flow ventriuclar assist device patients. The Journal of Heart Valve Disease. 2011;**20**(2):149-158

[52] Rose AG, Park SJ, Bank AJ, Miller LW. Partial aortic valve fusion induced by left ventricular assist device. The Annals of Thoracic Surgery. 2000;**70**(4):1270-1274

[53] Connelly J. Acquired commissural fusion of aortic valves in patients with left ventricular assist devices. The Journal of Heart and Lung Transplantation. 2003;**22**(12):1291-1295

[54] Kirklin JK, Pagani FD, Kormos RL, Stevenson LW, Blume ED, Myers SL,

et al. Eighth annual INTERMACS report: Special focus on framing the impact of adverse events. The Journal of Heart and Lung Transplantation. 2017;**36**(10):1080-1086

[55] Bouabdallaoui N, El-Hamamsy I, Pham M, Giraldeau G, Parent MC, Carrier M, et al. Aortic regurgitation in patients with a left ventricular assist device: A contemporary review. The Journal of Heart and Lung Transplantation. 2018;**37**(11):1289-1297

[56] Tilea I, Suciu H, Tilea B, Maria C, Ispas M, Constantin R. Anatomy and Function of Normal Aortic Valvular Complex. London, UK: Calcific Aortic Valve Disease. InTech; 2013

[57] Denolin H, Kuhn H, Krayenbuehl H, Loogen F, Reale A. The defintion of heart failure. European Heart Journal. 1983;**4**(7):445-448

[58] Walker GA, Masters KS, Shah DN, Anseth KS, Leinwand LA. Valvular Myofibroblast activation by transforming growth factor-β: Implications for pathological extracellular matrix remodeling in heart valve disease. Circulation Research. 2004;**95**(3):253-260

[59] Rajamannan NM, Evans FJ, Aikawa E, Grande-Allen KJ, Demer LL, Heistad DD, et al. Calcific aortic valve disease: Not simply a degenerative process: A review and agenda for research from the National Heart and lung and Blood institute aortic stenosis working group executive summary: Calcific aortic valve disease – 2011 update. Circulation. 2011;**124**(16):1783-1791

[60] Gharib M, Kremers D, Koochesfahani M, Kemp M. Leonardo's vision of flow visualization. Experiments in Fluids. 2002;**33**(1):219-223

[61] Fondard O, Detaint D, Iung B, Choqueux C, Adle-Biassette H, Jarraya M, et al. Extracellular matrix remodelling in human aortic valve disease: The role of matrix metalloproteinases and their tissue inhibitors. European Heart Journal. 2005;**26**(13):1333-1341

[62] Aikawa E, Aikawa M, Libby P, Figueiredo JL, Rusanescu G, Iwamoto Y, et al. Arterial and aortic valve calcification abolished by Elastolytic Cathepsin S deficiency in chronic renal disease. Circulation. 2009;**119**(13):1785-1794

[63] van Rijswijk JW, Vink A, Martina JR, Ramjankhan FZ, Goldschmeding R, de Jonge N, et al. Pathology of aortic valve remodeling after continuous-flow left ventricular assist device support. The Journal of Heart and Lung Transplantation. 2017;**36**(1):113-116

[64] Maurer G. Aortic regurgitation. Heart. 2006;**92**(7):994-1000

[65] Chaliki HP, Mohty D, Avierinos JF, Scott CG, Schaff HV, Tajik AJ, et al. Outcomes after aortic valve replacement in patients with severe aortic regurgitation and markedly reduced left ventricular function. Circulation. 2002;**106**(21):2687-2693

[66] Carabello BA. Vasodilators in aortic regurgitation — Where is the evidence of their effectiveness? The New England Journal of Medicine. 2005;**353**(13):1400-1402

[67] Nishimura RA, Otto CM, Bonow RO, Carabello BA, Erwin JP, Guyton RA, et al. 2014 AHA/ACC guideline for the Management of Patients with Valvular Heart Disease. Journal of the American College of Cardiology. 2014;**63**(22):e57-e185

[68] Nash PJ, Vitvitsky E, Li J, Cosgrove DM, Pettersson G, Grimm RA. Feasibility of valve repair for Regurgitant bicuspid aortic valves—An echocardiographic study. The Annals of Thoracic Surgery. 2005;**79**(5):1473-1479

[69] Robertson JO, Naftel DC, Meyers SL, Kirklin JK, Mertz GD, Prasad S, et al. Concomitant aortic valve procedures in patients undergoing implantation of continuous-flow LVADs: An INTERMACS database analysis. The Journal of Heart and Lung Transplantation. 2015;**34**(6):797-805

[70] Park SJ, Liao KK, Segurola R, Madhu KP, Miller LW. Management of aortic insufficiency in patients with left ventricular assist devices: a simple coaptation stitch method (Park's stitch). The Journal of Thoracic and Cardiovascular Surgery. 2004;**127**(1):264-266

[71] Adamson RM, Dembitsky WP, Baradarian S, Chammas J, May-Newman K, Chillcott S, et al. Aortic valve closure associated with HeartMate left ventricular device support: Technical considerations and long-term results. The Journal of Heart and Lung Transplantation. 2011;**30**(5):576-582

[72] Morgan JA, Brewer RJ. Modified central closure technique for treatment of aortic insufficiency in patients on left ventricular assist device support. ASAIO Journal. 2012;**58**(6):626-628

[73] Goda A, Takayama H, Pak SW, Uriel N, Mancini D, Naka Y, et al. Aortic valve procedures at the time of ventricular assist device placement. The Annals of Thoracic Surgery. 2011;**91**(3):750-754

[74] Savage EB, d'Amato TA, Magovern JA. Aortic valve patch closure: An alternative to replacement with HeartMate LVAS insertion. European Journal of Cardio-Thoracic Surgery. Sep 1999;**16**(3):359-361

[75] Estep JD, Stainback RF, Little SH, Torre G, Zoghbi WA. The role of echocardiography and other imaging modalities in patients with left ventricular assist devices. JACC: Cardiovascular Imaging. 2010;**3**(10):1049-1064

[76] Holtz J, Teuteberg J. Management of Aortic Insufficiency in the continuous flow left ventricular assist device population. Current Heart Failure Reports. 2014;**11**(1):103-110

Chapter 7

Perspective Chapter: The ProtekDuo® Cannula for Acute Mechanical Circulatory Support

Joseph M. Brewer, Ammar Sharif and Marc O. Maybauer

Abstract

The ProtekDuo® is a dual lumen cannula that can be used in numerous configurations to treat cardiogenic shock and hypotension. Its default function is as a temporary percutaneous right ventricular assist device (RVAD) system, however, other configurations both alone and with other mechanical circulatory support (MCS) devices have evolved. In addition to its use as a component of a ventricular assist device (VAD), it can be used as a cannula for extracorporeal membrane oxygenation (ECMO) and may serve as double lumen drainage cannula on cardiopulmonary bypass (CPB). The role of the cannula in ECMO has been described in multiple configurations including traditional veno-pulmonary (V-P) or "oxygenated RVAD" (oxyRVAD), veno-venopulmonary (V-VP), or venopulmonary-arterial (VP-A). This book chapter summarizes various configurations and technical aspects of the ProtekDuo(R) cannula in the management of hypotension and cardiogenic shock.

Keywords: cardiogenic shock, ECLS, ECMO, hypotension, right heart failure, Right Ventricular Assist Device (RVAD), ProtekDuo®

1. Introduction

Despite improved treatment and outcomes for many forms of cardiovascular disease, cardiogenic shock (CS) remains a common cause of mortality [1–3]. CS is classically recognized as a state of inadequate cardiac output, which if left uncorrected, may lead to tissue malperfusion and organ failure. Vasopressors and inotropes become necessary as conventional treatment options to maintain adequate organ perfusion [4].

Over the past decade, only marginal improvements have been noted in outcomes and mortality rates of CS. When complicated by acute myocardial infarction (AMI-CS), the mortality rate ranges from 50 to 60%, while mortality from acute decompensated heart failure-related CS is approximately 40% [5].

Whether due to impaired function of the right ventricle (RV), left ventricle (LV), or both, implementation of prompt medical management to correct low cardiac output and hypotension is necessary. However, when medical management fails, use of acute mechanical circulatory support (MCS) should be considered [2]. In this chapter, we focus on a particular device, the ProtekDuo® cannula, and its role in the management of patients with cardiogenic shock with acute RV failure. We also discuss its evolving roles in the treatment of LV and biventricular failure, both alone and in combination with other devices, as well as use in the treatment of combined cardiac and respiratory failure, which commonly co-exist in clinical practice.

2. Cardiogenic shock

Cardiogenic shock occurs most frequently as a result of acute myocardial infarction (MI) [6], though any disease process that impairs the functional capacity of the left ventricle (LV) or right ventricle (RV) can lead to cardiogenic shock [1]. For years, numerous definitions and clinical criteria for cardiogenic shock have existed [7–10], but in 2019 the Society for Cardiovascular Angiography & Interventions published a consensus statement on the classification of cardiogenic shock [2] that has been useful for assessment of patients as well as predicting outcomes [11]. In this consensus document, stages of cardiogenic shock are described based on physical exam findings, biochemical markers, and hemodynamic parameters [2]. A standardized, team-based approach to management of cardiogenic shock has been recommended due to the complexity of disease and number of treatment options [12]. Though a complete discussion of cardiogenic shock is beyond the scope of this chapter, a brief discussion of LV and RV failure follow.

2.1 Left ventricular failure

Numerous diseases can cause LV failure and cardiogenic shock though the most common are acute MI and acute decompensation of end-stage heart failure [3, 6]. In the setting of acute MI, there is impairment of regional myocardial contractility, which if significant, can become self-perpetuating as a result of further worsening coronary ischemia [6, 13]. Patients with chronic, end-stage heart failure may enter into an acutely decompensated state and progress to cardiogenic shock due to a number of factors including disease progression, medication or treatment non-adherence, or an acute cardiac insult [3]. Numerous other conditions can also lead to acute LV failure including, but not limited to, acute myocarditis, stress cardiomyopathy, and post-cardiotomy syndrome [13].

Management of cardiogenic shock with predominant LV failure begins with prompt recognition based on clinical criteria followed by a team-based approach to assessment including echocardiogram and hemodynamic values [12]. If acute MI is suspected or confirmed, a coronary angiogram should be performed with revascularization if able [13]. Patients are treated with inotropes and vasopressors to maintain adequate cardiac index and blood pressure. Failure to achieve goals with medications alone should prompt consideration of acute MCS [1, 12].

2.2 Right ventricular failure

Right ventricular failure is a complex clinical syndrome of fluid overload, low systolic function and cardiac output, and atrial or ventricular arrhythmias [14]. The two pathophysiologies of RV pressure and volume overload typically occur as a result of injury or stress and can occur alone or in combination to cause acute RV failure and reduced cardiac output [14, 15]. Acute rise in RV afterload can occur in the setting of acute pulmonary embolus or subacutely in the acute respiratory distress syndrome due to prolonged hypoxia and/or respiratory acidosis. Acute reductions in right ventricular contractility can occur from either ischemic etiology such as MI or from inflammatory etiologies such as myocarditis. Patients may also have chronic RV failure for which they are normally able to compensate yet may become acutely decompensated in the setting of additional increases in RV afterload or reduction in RV contractility [14, 16, 17].

Medical management of acute RV failure begins with fluid volume management, enhancing myocardial contractility, and optimizing RV afterload often with echocardiographic and pulmonary artery catheter (PAC) guidance [2, 13, 15, 17, 18]. Additionally, for patients with hypotension, peripheral vasopressors and inotropes may be required. If the shock state does not resolve with medical management, utilization of acute mechanical circulatory support (MCS) must be considered. Acute RV failure is a major cause of morbidity and mortality [17], thus timely evaluation and initiation of acute MCS is essential [15, 16].

Acute MCS can be used as a bridge to recovery for up to 75% of patients with acute RV failure [16], or if recovery is not possible, a bridge to durable assist devices or heart transplant. Multiple acute MCS devices capable of directly or indirectly bypassing the failed RV are available [16, 17]. In this chapter we will focus particularly on the ProtekDuo® cannula as a component of a right ventricular assist device (RVAD) system.

3. ProtekDuo® cannula

The ProtekDuo® is a single-site, dual-lumen cannula that is most commonly placed in the right internal jugular vein (IJV). When in its intended position, the cannula drains blood from its proximal ports in the right atrium and blood flow is directed through an extracorporeal circuit with or without oxygenator before being returned via the distal ports into the pulmonary artery. The cannula is available in two sizes, 29 and 31 French (Fr.) Placement in the IJV allows for ambulation of the patient. The percutaneous placement of this device has allowed it to be a less invasive support option in patients requiring mechanical (RV) support. See **Figure 1**.

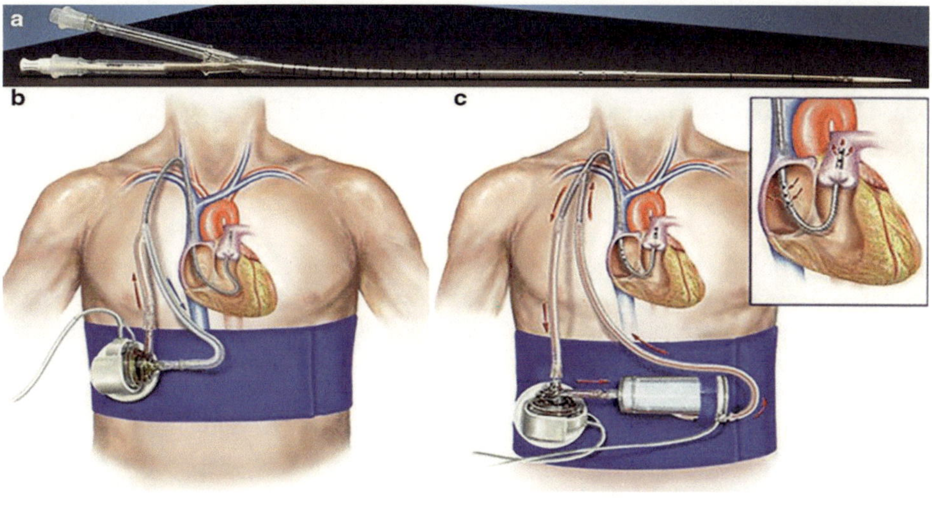

Figure 1.
a: Percutaneous right ventricular assist device (RVAD) with a Protek Duo cannula. b: Without oxygenator, and c: with oxygenator. From: Condello, I. Percutaneous right ventricular assist device, rapid employment in right ventricular failure during septic shock. Crit Care 24, 674 (2020).With kind permission from Critical Care (Open access).

3.1 ProtekDuo® cannulation technique

Placement of a ProtekDuo® involves use of the modified Seldinger technique. Initially the right IJV is assessed for adequate size and an 8-Fr to 9-Fr introducer sheath is placed. Using the sheath, a balloon tipped catheter is guided and placed into the right pulmonary artery (PA) under fluoroscopy. Then a long 0.035-inch Lunderquist Extra Stiff Wire Guide (Cook Medical, Denmark) is guided through the balloon tipped catheter under fluoroscopic guidance and inserted into the right PA. The balloon-tipped catheter is then removed carefully under fluoroscopic guidance to ensure that the stiff wire remains in place in the right PA. Then the neck sheath is removed, and the site is progressively dilated to a size below the size of the cannula being used. A heparin bolus, dosed to achieve an activated clotting time of 300 seconds is given and then the ProtekDuo® cannula is placed under continuous fluoroscopy with the goal of having the cannula outflow port in the main PA [19]. Alternative anticoagulation may be achieved with direct thrombin inhibitors (DTI) [20], such as argatroban [21] or bivalirudin [22].

Transesophageal echocardiography (TEE) is useful to verify position of the cannula in the PA if fluoroscopy is not available. Both ports are clamped and then a wet-to-wet connection is made with the drainage and return ports. Pump flow is increased per the clinician's discretion. The device is secured in place with a purse-string suture around the insertion site. Direct suturing to cannula body should be avoided as it may provoke erosion of the cannula wall. Suture rings are provided with the cannula which enable indirect fixation.

Once flow is initiated, a heparin or DTI infusion is initiated to maintain a partial thromboplastin time of 40-60 seconds, depending on the circuit used, which can later be adjusted to institutional protocols [19].

3.2 ProtekDuo® cannulation complications

There is limited data about ProtekDuo® related complications. Some authors have reported vascular injury during insertion, cannula thrombosis and cannula migration requiring repositing, but the occurrence of these seems to be low [23–26]. Additionally, there is also a case report about right coronary artery compression caused by the cannula which was resolved by repositioning [27] and a case series of superior vena cava syndrome in two patients [28].

3.3 Device weaning

Patients should be evaluated daily for readiness-to-wean from support with the ProtekDuo cannula® once myocardial recovery occurs in addition to improvement in hemodynamic parameters including [29, 30]. While no standardized protocol currently exists for device weaning, recommended strategies include incremental reduction of device flow by 0.5 L/min until flow is at 2 L/min [29, 30]. Once device flow is low, assessment of hemodynamic parameters as well as ventricular function by echocardiography and laboratory parameters such as lactate are performed [29, 30]. If needed, low doses of vasopressors or inotropes can be used to provide hemodynamic support [29]. If weaning parameters are acceptable, then device removal can be considered if appropriate [29, 30].

4. ProtekDuo® as a ventricular assist device

The ProtekDuo® cannula, when placed in the intended location and connected to an extracorporeal pump, is able to provide direct bypass of the RV. As clinicians have become more experienced with using the cannula, its use has been adapted to other situations where ventricular assistance is needed.

4.1 ProtekDuo® as an RVAD

In studies of RVADs as treatment for acute RV failure, survival has improved with earlier initiation of mechanical support [16, 23, 26, 31]. RVADs can be inserted surgically, via sternotomy or thoracotomy, or percutaneously. Most RVADs, especially the percutaneous type, are intended for temporary use. The ProtekDuo® cannula is a particularly advantageous component of a percutaneous RVAD system as it allows for expedient, upper body, percutaneous access with a single cannula, thus avoiding surgical implantation and explantation via sternotomy. See **Figure 1b**.

Use of the ProtekDuo® cannula as a component of an RVAD has been increasingly reported in the literature since its approval for use in humans in 2016. Retrospective cohort studies, case reports, and case series have described its use alone for isolated acute RV failure as well as in combination with a left ventricular assist device (LVAD) for biventricular support in the setting of concomitant left ventricular failure [23, 24, 26, 32–35].

4.1.1 ProtekDuo® for isolated acute RV failure

Acute RV failure can occur due to multiple etiologies including after temporary and durable left ventricular assist device (LVAD) implantation [23, 35], primary graft dysfunction after heart transplant [36], myocardial infarction [32], as well as other causes [24, 26, 33, 34].

Nicolais and colleagues [37] were among the first groups to report a larger series of patients with acute RV failure treated with the ProtekDuo®. In the series of 13 patients; four had acute myocardial infarction; three were bridge to lung or heart transplant; two had severe pulmonary hypertension; and one patient each had acute myocarditis, post-LVAD RV failure, or post-heart transplant graft dysfunction. The group reported a median duration of support of 6 days and 54% survival to device explantation. They concluded that the ProtekDuo® cannula could be used for short-term isolated RV support or in conjunction with a left ventricular support device for cases of biventricular failure while using single-site access [37].

Kremer et al. [32] conducted a retrospective study of 10 patients with acute myocardial infarction complication by acute RV failure who underwent ProtekDuo® implantation for RVAD support. Patients had significant reduction in right heart filling pressures and increase in cardiac output after device implantation. The mean duration of RVAD support with ProtekDuo® was 10 ± 7.4 days. The authors reported a 30-day and 1-year survival of 60% with four patients having complete recovery and two patients requiring placement of durable RVAD. A total of four patients required an interposed membrane oxygenator and there were no device-related complications. The authors concluded that the use of the ProtekDuo® cannula as a temporary RVAD was safe and feasible for patients with acute RV failure secondary to myocardial infarction [32].

Badu et al. [24] conducted a retrospective cohort study of 40 patients with acute RV failure grouped by primary cause: post-cardiotomy (n = 18), other cardiac causes including myocardial infarction and exacerbation of heart failure (n = 12), and severe respiratory failure (n = 10). The authors reported a significant reduction in vasopressor and inotrope requirements in all groups within 48 hours of device implantation. Device-related complications were reported including cannula migration in three patients, SVC syndrome in three patients, and right internal jugular vein thrombus in one patient. The authors reported duration of RVAD support with ProtekDuo® for patients who successfully weaned from support and patients who died on support. For patients who successfully weaned, the overall duration of support was a median of 14 days with patients in the post-cardiotomy group requiring support for a median of 15 days, other cardiac causes group 11 days, and respiratory failure group 10 days. For patients who died on support, the overall duration of support was a median of 5 days with patients in the post-cardiotomy group requiring support for a median of 43 days, other cardiac causes group 3 days, and respiratory failure group 15 days. The authors reported overall survival to discharge of 68% in the cohort. When survival to discharge was analyzed by cause of acute RV failure, the authors reported 89% survival in the post-cardiotomy group, 42% survival in the group of other cardiac causes, and 60% survival in the group with respiratory failure. The authors concluded that use of the ProtekDuo® cannula resulted in improved hemodynamics with reduced need for vasopressors and inotropes as well as high rates of weaning, low complications, and low mortality [24].

Oliveros and colleagues [34] conducted a retrospective study of 11 patients with acute RV failure from multiple causes including post-partum cardiomyopathy (with biventricular failure requiring simultaneous V-A ECMO support), following lung transplant, massive pulmonary embolism, myocardial infarction, and acute respiratory distress syndrome. The mean duration of RVAD support with ProtekDuo® was 58 ± 47 days. The authors reported 30-day survival of 82% and 180-day survival of 73%. The authors did not report device-related complications for the cohort [34].

Carrozzini et al. [36] reported a case series of three patients with acute RV failure due to primary graft dysfunction after heart transplant. Of note, all three patients required V-A ECMO prior to transplant due to end-stage biventricular failure. The authors reported complete unloading of the failed RV without distention of the LV by transesophageal echocardiogram. One patient experienced a right internal jugular vein thrombus. The patients required support from four to 12 days. All patients were successfully weaned and discharged alive. In treating these patients, the authors were able to avoid V-A ECMO or central right ventricular support. The authors concluded that the ProtekDuo® cannula was easy to insert, safe and effective and is the preferred temporary mechanical support device for patients with isolated RV primary graft dysfunction after heart transplant [36].

4.1.2 ProtekDuo® for biventricular failure

Biventricular shock is characterized by elevated CVP (>14 mmHg), normal or elevated PCWP (>18 mmHg) and hypotension, along with reduced LV function. At least 40% of patients diagnosed with LV-dominant CS, in fact have biventricular failure [5].

The use of temporary [38] and durable [39, 40] LVADs has continued to increase over the last decade. Acute RV failure after LVAD implantation is reported to occur in up to 40% of cases [26, 41–44]. Multiple causes, either alone or in combination, including unmasking of chronic RV dysfunction once RV preload increases, distortion of RV geometry due to bowing of the intraventricular septum toward the LV due to mechanical LV unloading, ventricular dysrhythmias, and embolic phenomenon to the coronary or pulmonary circulation are thought to precipitate RV failure [45]. Patients with LVADs who develop additional acute RV failure and require biventricular support have a high mortality [26].

Patients with shock in the setting of biventricular failure refractory to medical management are usually supported with V-A ECMO. However, if an LVAD is present, then the addition of isolated RV support can provide adequate cardiovascular support while avoiding potential challenges imposed by V-A ECMO including retrograde flow with increased LV afterload, complications of arterial access including extremity ischemia, and low transpulmonary flow [36]. The ProtekDuo® cannula may offer additional benefits including non-surgical, single-site access in the upper body, which may allow for earlier extubation and/or mobilization.

4.1.2.1 ProtekDuo® with temporary LVADs

A number of authors have presented cases of the ProtekDuo® cannula used in combination with an Impella temporary percutaneous LVAD for biventricular support. Our group has reported our experience with the combination of devices, which we describe using the novel portmanteau "PROpella" [46].

The Impella CP is a percutaneous LVAD capable of delivering up to 3.5 liters per minute of flow. Patel and colleagues reported a case of a patient with biventricular failure who was supported with the combination of a ProtekDuo® and Impella CP inserted via the axillary artery thus allowing the patient to be awake and ambulate. Chivasso et al. reported a case of a 38-year-old patient who underwent emergent coronary artery bypass grafting that was complicated by electrical storm initially supported with V-A ECMO, but was later converted to biventricular support with ProtekDuo® cannula and Impella CP. See **Figure 2**.

The Impella 5.0 (no longer available) and the newer Impella 5.5 are surgically placed and capable of delivering up to 5.5 liters per minute of flow. Routh and co-authors reported a case of a 61-year old man with inotrope-dependent nonischemic cardiomyopathy who developed acute cardiogenic shock initially treated with Impella 5.5. The patient subsequently developed acute RV failure and a ProtekDuo® cannula was placed, allowing for biventricular support [45]. Ramamurthi et al. reported a case series of six patients who underwent carotid placement of an Impella 5.5 for left ventricular support. One patient in the series, a 49-year-old woman, required placement of a ProtekDuo® cannula for concomitant RV failure. Care was later withdrawn due to inability to wean from mechanical support [47]. Kataria and colleagues described three cases of successful use of ProtekDuo® for acute right heart failure in patients with Impella 5.5 placed for heart failure-related cardiogenic shock, though specific outcomes of these patients were not discussed [48]. See **Figure 3**.

4.1.2.2 ProtekDuo® with durable LVADs

A number of authors have presented larger case series and retrospective cohort studies of patients supported with ProtekDuo® after implantation of durable LVAD.

Ravichandran and co-authors published a case series of 17 patients with acute RV failure supported with ProtekDuo® cannula. In their series, acute RV failure occurred mostly following implantation of an LVAD: 12 patients after durable LVAD implantation and one patient after temporary percutaneous LVAD implantation. The remaining four patients had acute RV failure due to other causes. Device-related

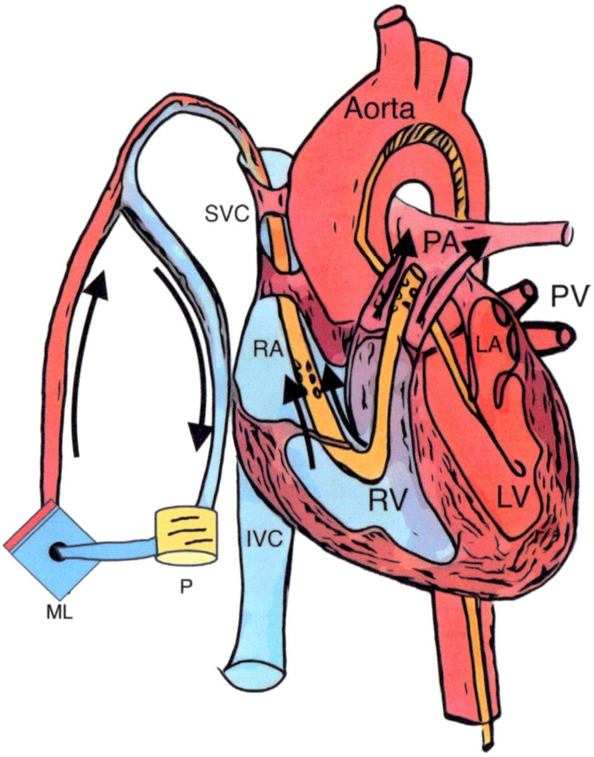

Figure 2.
PROpella approach with ProtekDuo® and oxygenator in RVAD/V-P ECMO position and Impella CP in LVAD position. Modified from: Maybauer MO et al. The ProtekDuo® in percutaneous peripheral venopulmonary-arterial ECMO and PROpella configuration for cardiogenic shock with biventricular failure. Ann Card Anaesth. In Press. With kind permission from Ann Card Anaesth.

complications including vessel injury occurred in one patient and bleeding from the cannula site in two patients. The mean duration of RVAD support with ProtekDuo® was 10.5 ± 6.5 days and six patients required conversion to surgical or durable RVAD for extended support [26].

In a retrospective study of 11 patients with acute RV failure at the time of durable LVAD implantation, Schmack et al. reported a mean duration of support with ProtekDuo® of 16.8 ± 9.5 days. The authors reported no device-related complications. In the series, 91% of patients survived to device weaning. The cohort had a 30-day survival of 73% and 180-day survival of 64% [35].

Salna and colleagues performed a retrospective study of 27 patients who underwent durable LVAD implantation and subsequently developed acute RV failure. All patients were placed on RVAD support using a ProtekDuo® cannula and were supported a median duration of 11 days. The median reported dose of required vasopressor and inotrope was significantly lower at 6-hours post-insertion. The authors reported an 85% survival to both discharge and at 30-days. Complications related to the ProtekDuo® cannula were few with cannula migration occurring in two patients and device-related thrombosis occurring in one patient. A total of three patients required conversion to surgical RVAD for prolonged support [23].

Lim and colleagues conducted a retrospective analysis of 11 patients with acute RV failure due to various etiologies. Most patients in the series had RV failure after LVAD:

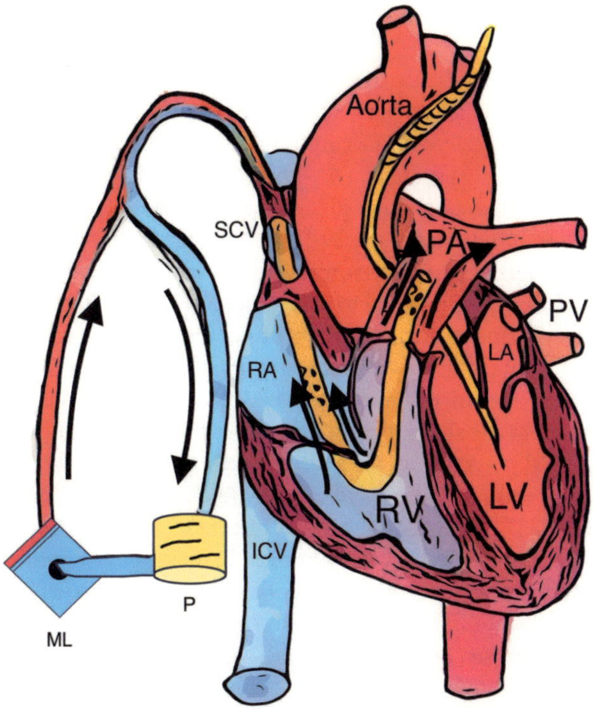

Figure 3.
PROpella approach with ProtekDuo® and oxygenator in RVAD/V-P ECMO position and Impella 5.5 in LVAD position. Modified from: Maybauer MO et al. The ProtekDuo® in percutaneous peripheral venopulmonary-arterial ECMO and PROpella configuration for cardiogenic shock with biventricular failure. Ann Card Anaesth. In Press. With kind permission from Ann Card Anaesth.

seven after durable LVAD and two with end-stage heart failure cardiogenic shock after temporary percutaneous LVAD implantation. The remaining two patients had post-heart transplant graft dysfunction. The authors reported a significant reduction in right heart filling pressures, but no significant difference in vasopressor and inotrope dose at 3-hours post-cannulation. The patients in this cohort required RVAD support with ProtekDuo® for a median duration of 10 days and had a 90-day survival of 64%. Device-related complications were not reported in this study [33].

4.2 ProtekDuo® as a left ventricular assist device

While uncommon, the ProtekDuo® cannula has also been used as an LVAD. Rao and colleagues described the use of a combined 21-Fr peripheral venous drainage cannula with a transapical 31-Fr ProtekDuo® cannula inserted via mini-thoracotomy for biventricular support in a 44-year-old with non-ischemic cardiomyopathy in cardiogenic shock [49]. Alaeddine and co-authors described the transapical placement of a 29-Fr ProtekDuo® cannula in a 10-year-old for temporary mechanical support prior to implantation of a total artificial heart [50]. Goodwin et al. described the use of a transapical 31-Fr ProtekDuo® cannula inserted via mini-thoracotomy for temporary left heart support in a 51-year-old patient with ischemic cardiomyopathy and cardiogenic shock, who was not expected to tolerate peripheral V-A ECMO due to significant aortic valve pathology [51].

4.3 ProtekDuo® as a biventricular assist device

Khalpey and colleagues first described the use of dual ProtekDuo® cannulas for biventricular support in three patients. The first patient was a 22-year-old with non-ischemic cardiomyopathy complicated by acute decompensated biventricular heart failure. The second patient was a 46-year-old with ischemic cardiomyopathy who underwent coronary artery stent placement with Impella support complicated by electrical storm. In both patients, a 29-Fr ProtekDuo® was modified and placed transapically into the left ventricle through a mini-thoracotomy followed by standard placement of a 29-Fr ProtekDuo® cannula in the pulmonary artery. This configuration allowed for extubation and ambulation of both patients until placement of total artificial heart while awaiting heart transplant in the first patient and recovery in the second patient. The third patient was a 63-year-old with anterior STEMI complicated by cardiogenic shock despite intra-aortic balloon counterpulsation. He underwent transapical placement of a ProtekDuo® cannula for LV support but had electrical storm and required placement of a ProtekDuo® cannula for RV support. The ProtekDuo® RVAD was weaned, but his family later consented to withdraw life support. The authors concluded that use of dual ProtekDuo® cannulas for biventricular support was a safe and effective method of establishing biventricular assist device (Bi-VAD) placement allowing avoidance of sternotomy, cardiopulmonary bypass with its associated complications, and peripheral ECMO while allowing for early extubation and ambulation [52].

5. The ProtekDuo® for extracorporeal membrane oxygenation

Conventional management for ARDS includes low tidal volume ventilation, neuromuscular blockage, and prone positioning. Pulmonary vasodilators are often used for temporary improvement of oxygenation and to bridge a patient to ECMO. Veno-venous (V-V) ECMO can be used in refractory hypoxemia and/or hypercapnia, or ventilator induced lung injury, and may typically be provided by single lumen dual site cannulation (femoro-internal jugular) or dual lumen single site cannulation (DLSC), typically via internal jugular vein approach. In the venous system, flow is dependent on the capacitance of the vessels, tricuspid competence, as well as systolic and diastolic function of both ventricles. In addition, pulmonary artery pressure, RV afterload, and total systemic cardiac output play an important role. V-V ECMO may display varying degrees of recirculation of blood depending on the flow rate, proximity of the inflow to outflow cannula(s), cannula location, and cannula size [53].

Impaired RV function occurs frequently in patients with ARDS [54, 55] and is associated with increased mortality [55, 56]. During the COVID-19 pandemic, clinicians observed a particularly high incidence of acute and subacute RV failure [57] with dramatic increases in pulmonary vascular resistance due to the combined effects of hypoxia, hypercapnia, lung injury, and attempted sedation weaning [58]. Additionally, hypercoagulation associated with COVID-19 frequently led to both macro- and micropulmonary emboli, which further increased pulmonary pressures, RV dilation, and failure of systolic pump function resulting in hypotension and need for inotropes and vasopressors [59]. Understanding RV biomechanics and, in particular, the relationship between the RV and PA is key to identifying different phases of RV dysfunction leading to RV failure, hypotension and death. ECMO cannulas bypassing the RV are now being increasingly utilized for COVID-19 ARDS to counterbalance RV dysfunction.

The ProtekDuo® dual lumen cannula is similar to other dual lumen cannulas and may be used for V-V ECMO in cases of ARDS. If significant RV dysfunction or failure is present and resulting in the requirement of inotropes and vasopressors to counterbalance hypotension, the cannula can be used for combined V-V ECMO and RV support, a configuration commonly referred to as V-P ECMO or oxyRVAD [60]. See **Figure 1c**. The main difference between the ProtekDuo® and other dual lumen cannulas is that the tip of the ProtekDuo® terminates in the main PA and not in the inferior vena cava as it is the case with other dual lumen cannulas. The ProtekDuo®'s V-P ECMO default position may be a particularly beneficial feature in ARDS, not only because it is able to bypass the RV, but because the area of venous blood drainage from the RA and area of oxygenated blood return in the main PA are separated by two cardiac valves (tricuspid and pulmonic valve) thus preventing recirculation, a phenomenon commonly seen with other dual lumen ECMO cannulas. Considering the length and diameter of the cannula, an average flow of 4.5 LPM may be achieved, which usually provides adequate blood flow and oxygenation [53].

The COVID 19 pandemic resulted in much longer ECMO run times than ECMO teams were accustomed to, the incidence of RV failure and hypotension increased because of prolonged ARDS with the development of some degree of pulmonary hypertension and the ProtekDuo® was used more frequently in V-P ECMO configuration, even as primary device to initiate ECMO. Several interesting configurations have been developed during the COVID-19 pandemic, mostly due to clinical desperation and medical necessity, as described below.

5.1 ProtekDuo® in V-P ECMO configuration

In a recent systematic review on the utilization of the Protek Duo cannula for V-P ECMO (**Figure 1c**) in ARDS secondary to COVID-19 infection, our group identified five suitable articles including 194 patients who underwent ProtekDuo® implantation in combination with an oxygenator. The ProtekDuo® demonstrated survival rates of 59–89% throughout the studies with a significant survival benefit [61].

Mustafa et al. presented their experience with the ProtekDuo® in V-P ECMO configuration for patients with ARDS secondary to COVID-19. The authors presented a case series of 40 patients with an average duration of mechanical ventilation of 13 days. They reported an 80 percent (32 patients) rate of successful ECMO weaning with a 73% (29 patients) survival rate [62].

Cain and colleagues compared 39 patients in a V-P ECMO group of 18 patients and an invasive mechanical ventilation (IMV) group of 21 patients. The authors displayed a significant reduction of in-hospital (52.4 vs. 11.1%, P = 0.0008) and 30-day mortality rates (42.9 vs. 5.6%, P = 0,011) in favor of the V-P ECMO group without complications related to the device. While the IMV group presented with 15 cases of acute kidney injury (AKI, 71.4%, P < 0.001), the V-P ECMO group did not display a single patient with AKI [63].

Saeed et al. compared the cannulation approach in a retrospective multicenter trial of 435 adult patients. They compared dual-site vs. single-site cannulation. For dual site they used the two most common approaches, femoral vein to femoral vein and femoral vein to internal jugular vein access. For the single site approach, they used either the Protek Duo, Crescent, or Avalon cannulas through an internal jugular vein. Out of 435 patients, 99 (23%) received the ProtekDuo®, 89 (20%) had single site inferior vena cava (IVC) approach, and 247 (57%) had dual site approach. The authors demonstrated that the 90-day in hospital mortality for the entire cohort was 55%. The unadjusted 90-day in hospital mortality was 60% for dual site, 41% for

ProtekDuo®, and 61% IVC approach. The 90-day in-hospital mortality was significantly lower in the ProtekDuo® group ($p = 0.029$), but not significantly different between single site IVC compared to dual site approach ($p = 0.86$). However, patients who were cannulated with the ProtekDuo® had longer duration of the ECMO runs compared to the other approaches but had shorter periods of mechanical ventilation and were more commonly discharged home [64].

A cohort of 54 patients was investigated by Smith and colleagues, comparing the ProtekDuo® with V-V ECMO for a one-year period during the pandemic. Thirty percent of their patients had V-V and 70% had V-P ECMO with a median time of 7 days from admission to ECMO cannulation. The authors reported a median ECMO support time of 30.5 days (V-V ECMO 35.0 days vs. V-P ECMO 26.0 days). Their mortality with V-P ECMO was 39.5%, with a 50.0% mortality for V-V ECMO with a total in-hospital mortality of 42.6%. The mortality after 120 days for V-V ECMO was 60.8% and only 40% for V-P ECMO, with a total cumulative mortality of 45.7%. This group concluded that ECMO support for ARDS secondary to COVID-19 is beneficial and that V-P ECMO support displayed consistent advantages in survival compared to V-V ECMO [65].

In addition to these studies, an interesting case was reported by Gianni et al., that may be very useful in patients with pulmonary embolism. In this patient, an inferior vena cava filter was positioned to prevent embolization from a left femoral deep venous thrombosis. The patient also had a large lesion of the tracheal posterior wall. Tracheal stenting required V-V ECMO support to safely perform the bronchoscopic procedure. Due to the presence of the inferior vena cava filter, the patient was cannulated with the ProtekDuo® cannula, since it does not interfere with the IVC, while dual site or double lumen cannulas typically end in the IVC. The patient could be weaned off ECMO after the procedure and the tracheal stent was removed after 40 days with full recovery, expanding the potential indications for the ProtekDuo® cannula [66].

5.2 Protek duo in V-VP ECMO configuration

This new technique and configuration for the ProtekDuo® was developed by Maybauer during the COVID-19 pandemic when treating a patient with persistent, severe hypoxia while on V-P ECMO with blood flows of 4.5 to 5 LPM. In an attempt to achieve more blood flow, a 25-Fr femoral multistage cannula was inserted for venous drainage. The post-pump tubing was spliced with a 3/8-in Y-connector to distribute the blood flow to both lumina of the ProtekDuo®, which resulted in return of oxygenated blood to the right atrium and main pulmonary artery in a configuration that could be best described as V-VP ECMO [67] (See **Figure 4**).

Returning blood flow improved to 7 LPM resulting in resolution of hypoxia and maintenance of $SpO2 > 90\%$, which finally allowed for the use of ventilator "rest settings" (Inspiratory Plateau Pressure < 25 to <30 cmH_2O, Respiration Rate 4-15 breaths per minute, PEEP >10 cmH_2O, FiO2 0.3 to 0.5). Using ultrasonic flow probes, blood flows to both ProtekDuo® lumina were measured and monitored independently. Due to length and diameter of the cannula, about 60% of flow returned into the RA and about 40% of flow returned into the pulmonary artery. Still, about 3 LPM bypassed the RV, which was sufficient to protect the RV in this patient. Frequently repeated transthoracic echocardiograms confirmed adequate decompression of the RV. The patient was able to separate from V-P-ECMO after 44 days with 29 days on the new configuration. The patient did not have any complications associated with this new configuration [67].

Most recently, the group of Maybauer presented a case series of nine patients, using the ProtekDuo® in V-P and V-VP ECMO configuration [19]. The authors could show

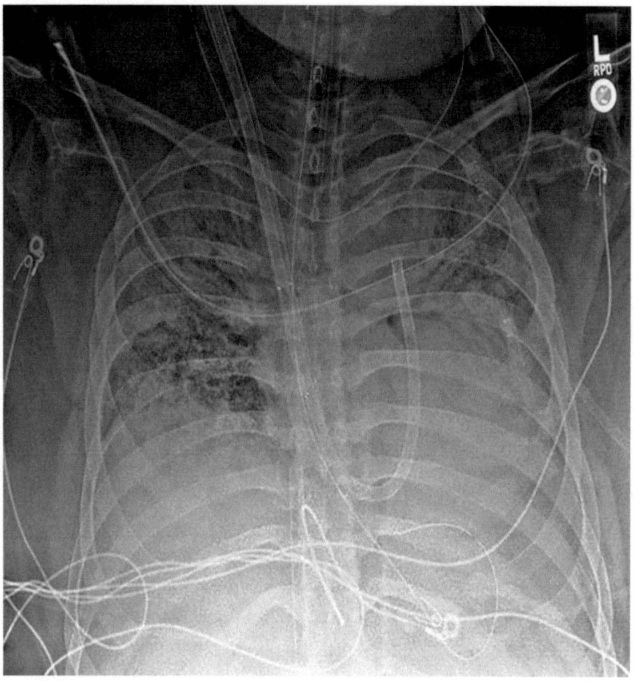

Figure 4.
Chest X-ray of ProtekDuo® in V-P ECMO position with additional 25Fr drainage cannula with tip in right atrial/inferior vena cava junction through a femoral vein. Drainage through the femoral cannula and return through both lumens of the ProtekDuo® using a Y-piece after the oxygenator. Modified from: Maybauer MO et al. The ProtekDuo® as double lumen return cannula in V-VP ECMO configuration: A first-in-man method description. Ann Card Anaesth. 2022;25(2):217-9. With kind permission from Ann Card Anaesth.

that in contrast to the above-mentioned studies where V-P ECMO was the initial configuration, this study showed that V-P or V-VP ECMO configuration was established weeks after the onset of ARDS with initial dual site V-V ECMO. This selected group of patients still displayed good outcomes with a survival rate of 67%, indicating the Protek Duo has been a game changer when used in patients with ARDS secondary to COVID-19 [68].

5.3 Protek duo in VP-A ECMO configuration

Budd et al., described the "central" VP-A ECMO configuration for a patient who was to receive a bilateral, sequential native pneumonectomy and donor lung transplantation after having V-P ECMO in situ. Following a sternotomy, they inserted an 18-Fr cannula (Edwards Lifesciences, Irvine, CA) into the ascending aorta. Thereafter, blood was drained through both lumens of the ProtekDuo® cannula and oxygenated blood was returned into the aorta as intraoperative central V-A ECMO configuration or more precisely called central VP-A configuration. After initiation, good decompression of the heart was achieved, which allowed for completion of pneumonectomy and donor lung transplantation. Before chest closure, the arterial cannula was removed and V-P ECMO was reinstated through the ProtekDuo® [69]. Similar techniques have been described by Settepani et al. for orthotopic heart transplantation [70] and by Sinha et al. in a combined heart and lung transplantation [71]. Either ECMO or cardiopulmonary bypass was used as pump in the above-mentioned circumstances of short intraoperative support.

Most recently, Maybauer et al. described a case with a patient who had a non ST elevation myocardial infarction (NSTEMI) and suffered a cardiac arrest on the catheter laboratory table. After return of spontaneous circulation (ROSC) was achieved, the patient developed biventricular failure with severe refractory hypotension and an Impella CP was placed. The patient remained in shock, requiring high doses of inotropes and vasopressors. A follow up echocardiogram demonstrated ongoing biventricular failure. A 29 Fr ProtekDuo® cannula was placed as RVAD with ECMO circuit in V-P configuration. With the Impella CP already in situ, a PROpella configuration was created (**Figure 2**), and the patient was stabilized. After a few hours, the patient displayed signs of limb ischemia due to occlusion of the femoral artery by the Impella CP. A thrombectomy and left calf fasciotomy was necessary and the Impella CP had to be removed. Because the patient developed pulmonary edema after Impella CP removal, a 17 French arterial and 5 Fr distal perfusion cannula were placed in the contralateral proximal femoral artery. The circuit tubing connected to the ProtekDuo® was clamped, cut, and wet connected to a new ECMO circuit using a Y-piece and used for dual-lumen venous drainage from both the RA and main PA. Oxygenated blood was returned through the 17-Fr arterial cannula, creating a "peripheral" VP-A ECMO configuration (**Figure 5**). This peripheral configuration

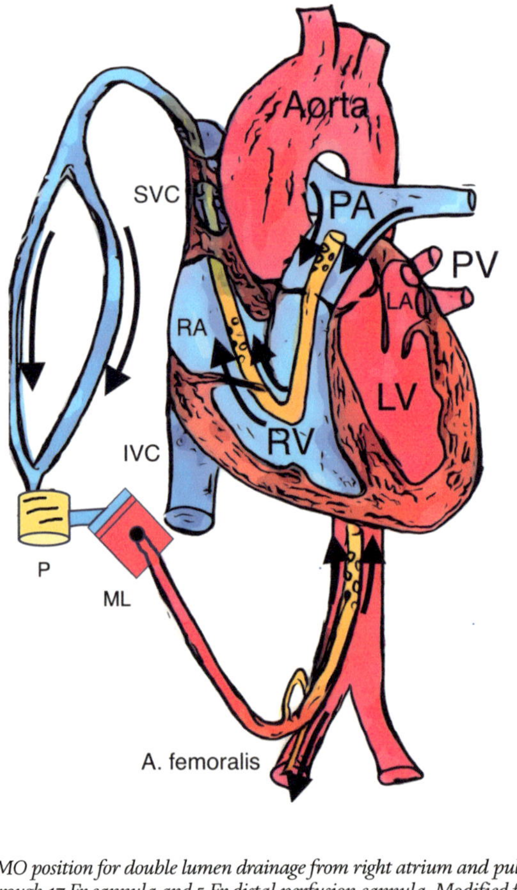

Figure 5.
ProtekDuo® in VP-A ECMO position for double lumen drainage from right atrium and pulmonary artery and return flow into femoral artery through 17 Fr cannula and 5 Fr distal perfusion cannula. Modified from: Maybauer MO et al. The ProtekDuo® in percutaneous peripheral venopulmonary-arterial ECMO and PROpella configuration for cardiogenic shock with biventricular failure. Ann Card Anaesth. In Press. With kind permission from Ann Card Anaesth.

however could be used for about 24 h without complications in comparison with the use of central VP-A configuration on CPB [46].

In a similar configuration, Kumar and colleagues described left ventricular unloading utilizing pulmonary artery drainage in cardiorespiratory failure due to COVID-19 infection. They described ProtekDuo® insertion for LV venting who was first on V-V ECMO and then converted to V-A and developed LV distention [72].

6. Conclusion

CS is a serious and life threating problem with high mortality rates. In case of acute ventricular failure, the main goal is to quickly implement measures to allow for ventricular recovery, by offloading volume and pressure, while maintaining adequate end-organ perfusion. When conventional treatment options fail, acute mechanical circulatory support is indicated. The ProtekDuo in RVAD configuration has the particular advantage over other single-site cannula-based temporary percutaneous RVADs because it is placed in the upper body versus the groin, thus allowing the patient to freely use the lower extremities in case of mobilization. Further, the ProtekDuo is compatible with a variety of blood pumps and may be used with a membrane oxygenator (ECMO) in case of concomitant respiratory failure, which is not an available option with other single-site, temporary percutaneous RVADs. When used in ECMO configuration, the ProtekDuo® may be used for V-P, V-VP, and VP-A ECMO as well as in PROpella configuration. Each option has specific benefits for patients requiring individual support for respiratory, right heart, left heart or biventricular failure. In V-P position, a mean blood flow of 4.5 LPM may be achieved but can be increased to 7 LPM in patients with V-VP configuration for ARDS. With increasing blood flow, increasing oxygenation may be achieved. Most literature on the ProtekDuo® in ARDS exists for COVID-19, where it has been shown to improve outcomes, reduce AKI and consecutively reduce the need for CRRT. The use of the ProtekDuo® for other ARDS etiologies has not yet been described. Cardiocirculatory support may be provided in PROpella or VP-A configuration. All options have been used and shown to be feasible. With a limited number of cases, safety cannot be guaranteed but may be likely.

Acknowledgements

The authors thank the Editor of Annals of Cardiac Anesthesia, Professor Mukul Chandra Kapoor, for kind permission to use figures from our previous publications in his journal, and LivaNova for covering the open access publication costs.

Conflict of interest

LivaNova covered the cost of publication. The authors have not received direct support.

Author details

Joseph M. Brewer[1], Ammar Sharif[1] and Marc O. Maybauer[2,3,4]*

1 Nazih Zuhdi Transplant Institute, Specialty Critical Care and Acute Circulatory Support, INTEGRIS Baptist Medical Center, Oklahoma City, OK, USA

2 Department of Anesthesiology, Division of Critical Care Medicine, University of Florida College of Medicine, Gainesville, FL, USA

3 Department of Anaesthesiology and Intensive Care Medicine, Philipps University, Marburg, Germany

4 Critical Care Research Group, The Prince Charles Hospital, The University of Queensland, Brisbane, Australia

*Address all correspondence to: mmaybauer@ufl.edu

References

[1] Vahdatpour C, Collins D, Goldberg S. Cardiogenic Shock. Journal of the American Heart Association. 2019;**8**(8):e011991

[2] Baran DA, Grines CL, Bailey S, Burkhoff D, Hall SA, Henry TD, et al. SCAI clinical expert consensus statement on the classification of cardiogenic shock: This document was endorsed by the American College of Cardiology (ACC), the American Heart Association (AHA), the Society of Critical Care Medicine (SCCM), and the Society of Thoracic Surgeons (STS) in April 2019. Catheterization and Cardiovascular Interventions. 2019;**94**(1):29-37

[3] Abraham J, Blumer V, Burkhoff D, Pahuja M, Sinha SS, Rosner C, et al. Heart failure-related cardiogenic shock: pathophysiology, evaluation and management considerations: Review of heart failure-related cardiogenic shock. Journal of Cardiac Failure. 2021;**27**(10):1126-1140

[4] Basir MB, Schreiber T, Dixon S, Alaswad K, Patel K, Almany S, et al. Feasibility of early mechanical circulatory support in acute myocardial infarction complicated by cardiogenic shock: The Detroit cardiogenic shock initiative. Catheterization and Cardiovascular Interventions. 2018;**91**(3):454-461

[5] Atti V, Narayanan MA, Patel B, Balla S, Siddique A, Lundgren S, et al. A comprehensive review of mechanical circulatory support devices. Heart International. 2022;**16**(1):37-48

[6] Samsky MD, Morrow DA, Proudfoot AG, Hochman JS, Thiele H, Rao SV. Cardiogenic shock after acute myocardial infarction: A review. Journal of the American Medical Association. 2021;**326**(18):1840-1850

[7] Stevenson LW, Pagani FD, Young JB, Jessup M, Miller L, Kormos RL, et al. INTERMACS profiles of advanced heart failure: The current picture. The Journal of Heart and Lung Transplantation. 2009;**28**(6):535-541

[8] Hochman JS, Sleeper LA, Webb JG, Sanborn TA, White HD, Talley JD, et al. Early revascularization in acute myocardial infarction complicated by cardiogenic shock. SHOCK Investigators. Should We Emergently Revascularize Occluded Coronaries for Cardiogenic Shock. The New England Journal of Medicine. 1999;**341**(9):625-634

[9] Ponikowski P, Voors AA, Anker SD, Bueno H, Cleland JGF, Coats AJS, et al. 2016 ESC Guidelines for the diagnosis and treatment of acute and chronic heart failure: The Task Force for the diagnosis and treatment of acute and chronic heart failure of the European Society of Cardiology (ESC)Developed with the special contribution of the Heart Failure Association (HFA) of the ESC. European Heart Journal. 2016;**37**(27):2129-2200

[10] Thiele H, Zeymer U, Neumann FJ, Ferenc M, Olbrich HG, Hausleiter J, et al. Intraaortic balloon support for myocardial infarction with cardiogenic shock. The New England Journal of Medicine. 2012;**367**(14):1287-1296

[11] Naidu SS, Baran DA, Jentzer JC, Hollenberg SM, van Diepen S, Basir MB, et al. SCAI SHOCK stage classification expert consensus update: A review and incorporation of validation studies: This statement was endorsed by the American College of Cardiology (ACC), American College of Emergency

Physicians (ACEP), American Heart Association (AHA), European Society of Cardiology (ESC) Association for Acute Cardiovascular Care (ACVC), International Society for Heart and Lung Transplantation (ISHLT), Society of Critical Care Medicine (SCCM), and Society of Thoracic Surgeons (STS) in December 2021. Journal of the American College of Cardiology. 2022;**79**(9):933-946

[12] Tehrani BN, Truesdell AG, Sherwood MW, Desai S, Tran HA, Epps KC, et al. Standardized team-based care for cardiogenic shock. Journal of the American College of Cardiology. 2019;**73**(13):1659-1669

[13] van Diepen S, Katz JN, Albert NM, Henry TD, Jacobs AK, Kapur NK, et al. Contemporary management of cardiogenic shock: A scientific statement from the american heart association. Circulation. 2017;**136**(16):e232-ee68

[14] Haddad F, Doyle R, Murphy DJ, Hunt SA. Right ventricular function in cardiovascular disease, part II: Pathophysiology, clinical importance, and management of right ventricular failure. Circulation. 2008;**117**(13):1717-1731

[15] Harjola VP, Mebazaa A, Celutkiene J, Bettex D, Bueno H, Chioncel O, et al. Contemporary management of acute right ventricular failure: A statement from the heart failure association and the working group on pulmonary circulation and right ventricular function of the european society of cardiology. European Journal of Heart Failure. 2016;**18**(3):226-241

[16] Konstam MA, Kiernan MS, Bernstein D, Bozkurt B, Jacob M, Kapur NK, et al. Evaluation and management of right-sided heart failure: A scientific statement from the american heart association. Circulation. 2018;**137**(20):e578-e622

[17] Kapur NK, Esposito ML, Bader Y, Morine KJ, Kiernan MS, Pham DT, et al. Mechanical circulatory support devices for acute right ventricular failure. Circulation. 2017;**136**(3):314-326

[18] Ranka S, Mastoris I, Kapur NK, Tedford RJ, Rali A, Acharya P, et al. Right heart catheterization in cardiogenic shock is associated with improved outcomes: insights from the nationwide readmissions database. Journal of the American Heart Association. 2021;**10**(17):e019843

[19] El Banayosy AM, El Banayosy A, Brewer JM, Mihu MR, Chidester JM, Swant LV, et al. The ProtekDuo for percutaneous V-P and V-VP ECMO in patients with COVID-19 ARDS. The International Journal of Artificial Organs. 2022;**45**(12):1006-1012

[20] Geli J, Capoccia M, Maybauer DM, Maybauer MO. Direct thrombin inhibition in extracorporeal membrane oxygenation. The International Journal of Artificial Organs. 2022;**45**(7):652-655

[21] Geli J, Capoccia M, Maybauer DM, Maybauer MO. Argatroban anticoagulation for adult extracorporeal membrane oxygenation: A systematic review. Journal of Intensive Care Medicine. 2022;**37**(4):459-471

[22] Sanfilippo F, Asmussen S, Maybauer DM, Santonocito C, Fraser JF, Erdoes G, et al. Bivalirudin for alternative anticoagulation in extracorporeal membrane oxygenation: A systematic review. Journal of Intensive Care Medicine. 2017;**32**(5):312-319

[23] Salna M, Garan AR, Kirtane AJ, Karmpaliotis D, Green P, Takayama H, et al. Novel percutaneous dual-lumen

cannula-based right ventricular assist device provides effective support for refractory right ventricular failure after left ventricular assist device implantation. Interactive Cardiovascular and Thoracic Surgery. 2020;**30**(4):499-506

[24] Badu B, Cain MT, Durham LA 3rd, Joyce LD, Sundararajan S, Gaglianello N, et al. A dual-lumen percutaneous cannula for managing refractory right ventricular failure. ASAIO Journal. 2020;**66**(8):915-921

[25] Agrawal N, Hameed F, Battel L, Arora A, Kumar S, Akkanti B, et al. Clinical outcomes in acute right ventricular failure with percutaneous right ventricular assist devices: Impella RP and Protek Duo. Journal of the American College of Cardiology. 2021;**77**(18 Supplement 1):634

[26] Ravichandran AK, Baran DA, Stelling K, Cowger JA, Salerno CT. Outcomes with the Tandem Protek duo dual-lumen percutaneous right ventricular assist device. ASAIO Journal. 2018;**64**(4):570-572

[27] Unger ED, Sweis RN, Bharat A. Unusual complication of a right ventricular support-extracorporeal membrane oxygenation cannula. JAMA Cardiology. 2021;**6**(6):723-724

[28] Badu B, Durham L 3rd, Joyce LD, Joyce DL. Iatrogenic superior vena cava syndrome from percutaneous right ventricular assist device. JTCVS Technology. 2021;**6**:92-94

[29] Geller BJ, Sinha SS, Kapur NK, Bakitas M, Balsam LB, Chikwe J, et al. Escalating and de-escalating temporary mechanical circulatory support in cardiogenic shock: A scientific statement from the american heart association. Circulation. 2022;**146**(6):e50-e68

[30] Randhawa VK, Al-Fares A, Tong MZY, Soltesz EG, Hernandez-Montfort J, Taimeh Z, et al. A pragmatic approach to weaning temporary mechanical circulatory support: A state-of-the-art review. JACC Heart Failure. 2021;**9**(9):664-673

[31] Coromilas EJ, Takeda K, Ando M, Cevasco M, Green P, Karmpaliotis D, et al. Comparison of percutaneous and surgical right ventricular assist device support after durable left ventricular assist device insertion. Journal of Cardiac Failure. 2019;**25**(2):105-113

[32] Kremer J, Farag M, Brcic A, Zubarevich A, Schamroth J, Kreusser MM, et al. Temporary right ventricular circulatory support following right ventricular infarction: Results of a groin-free approach. ESC Heart Failure. 2020;**7**(5):2853-2861

[33] Lim HS, Ranasinghe A, Mascaro J. The physiology of percutaneous right ventricular assist device-potential effects on ventilation-perfusion matching. ASAIO Journal. 2020;**66**(2):e31-ee2

[34] Oliveros E, Collado FM, Poulin MF, Seder CW, March R, Kavinsky CJ. Percutaneous right ventricular assist device using the tandemheart protekduo: Real-world experience. The Journal of Invasive Cardiology. 2021;**33**(6):E407-EE11

[35] Schmack B, Farag M, Kremer J, Grossekettler L, Brcic A, Raake PW, et al. Results of concomitant groin-free percutaneous temporary RVAD support using a centrifugal pump with a double-lumen jugular venous cannula in LVAD patients. Journal of Thoracic Disease. 2019;**11**(Suppl. 6):S913-SS20

[36] Carrozzini M, Merlanti B, Olivieri GM, Lanfranconi M, Bruschi G,

Mondino M, et al. Percutaneous RVAD with the Protek Duo for severe right ventricular primary graft dysfunction after heart transplant. The Journal of Heart and Lung Transplantation. 2021;**40**(7):580-583

[37] Nicolais CD, Suryapalam M, O'Murchu B, Bashir R, O'Neill BP, Alvarez R, et al. Use of Protek Duo Tandem Heart for percutaneous right ventricular support in various clinical settings: A case series. Journal of the American College of Cardiology. 2018;**71**(11 Supplement):A1314

[38] Vallabhajosyula S, Arora S, Lahewala S, Kumar V, Shantha GPS, Jentzer JC, et al. Temporary mechanical circulatory support for refractory cardiogenic shock before left ventricular assist device surgery. Journal of the American Heart Association. 2018;**7**(22):e010193

[39] Varshney AS, DeFilippis EM, Cowger JA, Netuka I, Pinney SP, Givertz MM. Trends and outcomes of left ventricular assist device therapy: JACC focus seminar. Journal of the American College of Cardiology. 2022;**79**(11):1092-1107

[40] Briasoulis A, Inampudi C, Akintoye E, Adegbala O, Alvarez P, Bhama J. Trends in utilization, mortality, major complications, and cost after left ventricular assist device implantation in the United States (2009 to 2014). The American Journal of Cardiology. 2018;**121**(10):1214-1218

[41] Anderson M, Morris DL, Tang D, Batsides G, Kirtane A, Hanson I, et al. Outcomes of patients with right ventricular failure requiring short-term hemodynamic support with the Impella RP device. The Journal of Heart and Lung Transplantation. 2018;**37**(12):1448-1458

[42] Lo Coco V, De Piero ME, Massimi G, Chiarini G, Raffa GM, Kowalewski M, et al. Right ventricular failure after left ventricular assist device implantation: A review of the literature. Journal of Thoracic Disease. 2021;**13**(2):1256-1269

[43] Kang G, Ha R, Banerjee D. Pulmonary artery pulsatility index predicts right ventricular failure after left ventricular assist device implantation. The Journal of Heart and Lung Transplantation. 2016;**35**(1):67-73

[44] Fida N, Loebe M, Estep JD, Guha A. Predictors and management of right heart failure after left ventricular assist device implantation. Methodist DeBakey Cardiovascular Journal. 2015;**11**(1):18-23

[45] Routh S, Fabrizio C, Sciortino CM, Kilic A, Toma C, Ramanan R, et al. Acute right ventricular failure in a patient with nonischemic cardiogenic shock on left-sided mechanical circulatory support. Journal of Cardiac Surgery. 2021;**36**(10):3884-3888

[46] Maybauer MO, Swol J, Sharif A, Benson C, Brewer JM. The ProtekDuo in percutaneous peripheral venopulmonary-arterial ECMO and PROpella configuration for cardiogenic shock with biventricular failure. Annals of Cardiac Anaesthesia. In Press

[47] Ramamurthi A, Cain MT, Smith N, Espinal A, Joyce DL, Mohammed A, et al. Transcarotid approach to placement of an impella 5.0. ASAIO Journal. 2022;**68**(1):e12-ee5

[48] Kataria R, Khalil A, Coglianese E, Crowley J, Silverman MG, Shelton K, et al. Effect of Impella 5.5 on preexisting functional mitral regurgitation in patients with heart failure–Related cardiogenic shock. Struct Heart. 2022;**6**(4):100072

[49] Rao P, Alouidor B, Smith R, Khalpey Z. Ambulatory central VA-ECMO with biventricular decompression for acute cardiogenic shock. Catheterization and Cardiovascular Interventions. 2018;**92**(5):1002-1004

[50] Alaeddine M, Ploutz M, Arabia FA, Velez DA. Implantation of total artificial heart in a 10-year-old after support with a temporary perventricular assist device. The Journal of Thoracic and Cardiovascular Surgery. 2020;**159**(3):e227-e2e9

[51] Goodwin ML, Roberts S, Lampert BC, Whitson BA. Temporary extracorporeal left ventricular support with transapical ProtekDuo cannula. JTCVS Technology. 2021;**5**:76-79

[52] Khalpey Z, Smith R, Echeverria A, le Tran P, Kazui T. A novel minimally invasive off-pump biventricular assist device insertion technique. The Journal of Thoracic and Cardiovascular Surgery. 2016;**151**(1):e5-e7

[53] Maybauer MO, Koerner MM, Swol J, El Banayosy A, Maybauer DM. The novel ProtekDuo ventricular assist device: Configurations, technical aspects, and present evidence. Perfusion. 2022:2676591221090607

[54] Petit M, Jullien E, Vieillard-Baron A. Right ventricular function in acute respiratory distress syndrome: Impact on outcome, respiratory strategy and use of veno-venous extracorporeal membrane oxygenation. Frontiers in Physiology. 2021;**12**:797252

[55] Zochios V, Parhar K, Tunnicliffe W, Roscoe A, Gao F. The right ventricle in ARDS. Chest. 2017;**152**(1):181-193

[56] Sato R, Dugar S, Cheungpasitporn W, Schleicher M, Collier P, Vallabhajosyula S, et al. The impact of right ventricular injury on the mortality in patients with acute respiratory distress syndrome: A systematic review and meta-analysis. Critical Care. 2021;**25**(1):172

[57] Paternoster G, Bertini P, Innelli P, Trambaiolo P, Landoni G, Franchi F, et al. Right ventricular dysfunction in patients With COVID-19: A systematic review and meta-analysis. Journal of Cardiothoracic and Vascular Anesthesia. 2021;**35**(11):3319-3324

[58] Argulian E, Sud K, Vogel B, Bohra C, Garg VP, Talebi S, et al. Right ventricular dilation in hospitalized patients with COVID-19 infection. JACC: Cardiovascular Imaging. 2020;**13**(11):2459-2461

[59] Corica B, Marra AM, Basili S, Cangemi R, Cittadini A, Proietti M, et al. Prevalence of right ventricular dysfunction and impact on all-cause death in hospitalized patients with COVID-19: A systematic review and meta-analysis. Scientific Reports. 2021;**11**(1):17774

[60] Condello I. Percutaneous right ventricular assist device, rapid employment in right ventricular failure during septic shock. Critical Care. 2020;**24**(1):674

[61] Maybauer MO, Capoccia M, Maybauer DM, Lorusso R, Swol J, Brewer JM. The ProtekDuo in ECMO configuration for ARDS secondary to COVID-19: A systematic review. The International Journal of Artificial Organs. 2022;**46**(2):93-98

[62] Mustafa AK, Alexander PJ, Joshi DJ, Tabachnick DR, Cross CA, Pappas PS, et al. Extracorporeal membrane oxygenation for patients With COVID-19 in severe respiratory failure. JAMA Surgery. 2020;**155**(10):990-992

[63] Cain MT, Smith NJ, Barash M, Simpson P, Durham LA 3rd, Makker H, et al. Extracorporeal membrane oxygenation with right ventricular assist device for COVID-19 ARDS. The Journal of Surgical Research. 2021;**264**:81-89

[64] Saeed O, Stein LH, Cavarocchi N, Tatooles AJ, Mustafa A, Jorde UP, et al. Outcomes by cannulation methods for venovenous extracorporeal membrane oxygenation during COVID-19: A multicenter retrospective study. Artificial Organs. 2022;**46**(8):1659-1668

[65] Smith NJ, Park S, Zundel MT, Dong H, Szabo A, Cain MT, et al. Extracorporeal membrane oxygenation for COVID-19: An evolving experience through multiple waves. Artificial Organs. 2022;**46**(11):2257-2265

[66] Giani M, Pisa A, Passera E, Avalli L, Rona R, Foti G. Tracheal stenting on venovenous ECMO with a dual lumen right atrium-to-pulmonary artery cannula in a COVID-19 patient with an inferior vena cava filter. Perfusion. 2022;**38**(3):654-656

[67] Maybauer MO, Koerner MM, Mihu MR, Harper MD, El Banayosy A. The ProtekDuo as double lumen return cannula in V-VP ECMO configuration: A first-in-man method description. Annals of Cardiac Anaesthesia. 2022;**25**(2):217-219

[68] Maybauer MO, Lorusso R, Swol J. The ProtekDuo cannula for extracorporeal membrane oxygenation: A game changer in COVID-19! Artificial Organs. 2022;**46**(11):2107-2108

[69] Budd AN, Kozarek K, Kurihara C, Bharat A, Reynolds A, Kretzer A. Use of ProtekDuo as veno-arterial and veno-venous extracorporeal membrane oxygenation during bilateral lung transplantation. Journal of Cardiothoracic and Vascular Anesthesia. 2019;**33**(8):2250-2254

[70] Settepani F, Marianeschi SM, Costetti A, Russo CF. Switch from minimally invasive biventricular mechanical support to cardiopulmonary bypass during heart transplant. European Journal of Cardio-Thoracic Surgery. 2021;**59**(1):271-273

[71] Sinha N, Goodarzi A, Akku R, Balayla G. ProtekDuo as a bridge to lung transplant and heart-lung transplant. Clinical Transplantation. 2021;**35**(5):e14273

[72] Kumar K, Coonse K, Zakhary B, Cigarroa JE. Novel method for left ventricular unloading utilizing percutaneous pulmonary artery drainage in cardiorespiratory failure due to COVID-19 infection. Catheterization and Cardiovascular Interventions. 2022;**100**(1):175-178

Section 5

Delivery of Mechanical Circulatory Support Care to Remote Communities

Chapter 8

Perspective Chapter: Delivering LVAD Care to the Local Community

Michael Sobieraj, Antonio Valone, Brisha Bhikadiya, Ricardo Chia and Kulpreet Barn

Abstract

Heart failure is a growing pandemic affecting approximately 6.2 million people in the US and 15 million people worldwide. Mechanical circulatory support devices are not only a bridge to transplantation, but have become destination therapy for a large portion of this population. Given its prevalence and high morbidity and mortality leading to significant financial burden on our healthcare system, establishing strategies focused on improving therapeutic outcomes and prognosis should be prioritized. Delivering care to such a large and complex patient population poses unique challenges given the progressive care needs and extensive follow-up. Time and distance traveled are among the limiting factors that disable patients from having access to life sustaining advanced therapies such as the LVAD. This chapter aims to review the traditional care model and expand on the necessary tools and benefits of the LVAD shared care model in delivering care to previously underserved patient populations with advanced heart failure.

Keywords: LVAD, destination therapy, shared care, outcomes, satisfaction

1. Introduction

Heart failure (HF) is a condition with high mortality due to decreased cardiac function leading to poor perfusion, exacerbated during high metabolic states. It is a growing pandemic expected to rise by almost 30%, expanding its reach from 6.2 million to 8 million people by 2030 in the US and many more worldwide [1–3]. It carries significant morbidity and dramatically limits patients' quality of life. The morbidity is costly, leading to high expenditures of 30.7 billion dollars annually, which is also projected to double by 2030 [4, 5]. The symptoms are debilitating as the disease progresses towards its end stages of advanced heart failure (AdHF) even despite maximally tolerated guideline directed medical therapy. At this stage in the disease process, medical therapy is inadequate and treatment must be advanced to more invasive means [6, 7]. The only viable options are orthotopic heart transplant or durable mechanical support in the form of a left ventricular assist device (LVAD). As the therapy advances, the treatment team must adapt to a multidisciplinary cohort incorporating a multitude of care providers from varying backgrounds [8–10].

IntechOpen

Few places have the resources capable of staffing such a diversity of providers, which comes at great expense, therefore traditionally limiting care to large academic centers. Patients that do not live near these centers face geographic barriers to care coordination and are prohibited from otherwise appropriate life prolonging care. The new shared care model allows for device implantation at a large center with the subsequent transfer of follow up care to a local heart failure program capable of managing LVAD recipients. This concept allows for greater access and thereby increases effective eligibility for advanced therapies. It also improves patient adherence to the rigorous home care regimens that LVADs require. Improved access and adherence ultimately improves patient outcomes and reduces their financial burden [11].

2. Advancing therapies

Worldwide, there are an increasing number of end stage heart failure patients with LVADs which now exceeds 100,000 of which 18,539 are reported in the Interagency Registry for Mechanically Assisted Circulatory Support (Intermacs) [5, 12] and 16,286 reported in the global IMACS registry collecting data from the United States, Europe, Japan, and United Kingdom [13]. As the end-stage heart failure pandemic continues to grow and alter the lives of multiple patients, LVAD advancements provide a viable option for patients as either a bridge to heart transplant or as destination therapy for those who are not transplant candidates.

MOMENTUM 3 is a landmark multicenter trial demonstrating the strides in LVAD technologies and decreasing patient complication rates. The centrifugal-flow LVAD, HeartMate III, demonstrated superior performance to the axial-flow LVAD, HeartMate II. The HeartMate III reduces shear stress, reduces friction, and prevents thrombosis. The primary outcome of the MOMENTUM 3 trial showed that 74.7% of patients with a HeartMate III survived without disabling stroke or reoperation to replace or remove a malfunctioning device at 2 years versus 60.6% of patients with the HeartMate II. Secondary outcomes of the study revealed decreased pump thrombosis, stroke, and bleeding events in the HeartMate III compared to the HeartMate II. The 3 year survival rate when utilizing HeartMate III now rivals that of heart transplantation [14]. This allows LVADs to extend life-prolonging therapy to patients not eligible for heart transplant and give patients an option that they never had before. The prevalence of adHF and life prolonging impact of LVADs worldwide makes the further development of LVAD care networks a pivotal part of delivering adHF care and improving patient outcomes.

3. Traditional LVAD care model

In traditional advanced heart failure centers, the care for these patients was provided by large multidisciplinary teams involving multiple coordinators, nurses, physician assistants, cardiothoracic surgeons, palliative care, and various advanced heart failure specialists. Due to the costs associated with such a large team, LVAD care was historically limited to large, urban medical facilities [15, 16]. Post-transplantation inpatient cardiac rehabilitation allows patients to improve their functional status. This also allowed for adjustment of LVAD settings as vital signs fluctuated with the body's adjustment to altered hemodynamics. Since patients with LVADs do not have a true systolic blood pressure, their mean arterial pressure (MAP) can be measured with a portable doppler by a trained professional. In addition to the vital signs, the degree of anticoagulation requires close monitoring as early data suggests that direct oral acting agents carry an increased risk of thrombotic events [17–19].

Patients and caregivers are required to attend extensive educational sessions at all LVAD implantation centers. These sessions evaluate patients' functional status in an effort to avoid catastrophic errors while performing daily care such as changing batteries, bathing, or responding to device alarms [20]. Training the patients to manage the driveline using sterile technique is extensive. Standardized kits have been generated to aid in the process, but driveline site infections remain a major concern and a cumbersome task for the patient [11, 21]. Driveline care requires significant adjustment to lifestyle, including intimate relationships. Patients are directed to be exceedingly careful to avoid pressure on equipment or excessive body movements near the exit site [22]. Similar to other major cardiac surgeries, after appropriate rehabilitation and wound healing, driving is permitted. Traveling requires additional preparation to ensure back ups to all equipment is available along with a LVAD site at destination [23].

While a multidisciplinary team optimizes care of an LVAD patient, a recent national survey of cardiologists, LVAD advanced practice providers, coordinators, surgeons, and social workers failed to identify the characteristics that would make an ideal patient [24]. Patients with higher education levels (>12 years) had higher survival rates [25]. The Singapore LVAD program has stricter selection criteria, however, the program's outcomes were similar to the IMACS registry. They did report a higher 3 year survival, but also a higher infection rate [26].

LVAD patients are frequently hospitalized due to complications with as many as 80% of all patients having had at least one admission by the 1 year mark [11]. Most commonly, they present with gastrointestinal bleeding (GIB) or a driveline infection. Optimal social support and meticulous adherence to LVAD management have been noted in conjunction with reduction in unplanned admissions. In 2020, there was a case report noting 4 years as the longest time interval to hospitalization for an LVAD patient. University of Chicago has conducted many trials investigating the infrastructure leading to LVAD success. They suggest the continuation of GDMT to decrease HF recurrence, omega-3 to decrease GIB [27, 28], bi-monthly international normalized ratio (INR) checks to maintain therapeutic anticoagulation [29], and a coordinator team to address all device alarms as measures to prevent adverse events and related unplanned readmissions [30]. The Miami Transplant Institute conducted a CF-LVAD study which showed anticoagulation management by a pharmacist along with self-testing improved the duration of time spent in therapeutic range [31]. With advancing technology, telehealth may serve as an adjunct to improving patient care. A small study utilizing a LVAD specific platform where patients entered their parameters followed by health surveys improved patient satisfaction. This platform gives patients the ability to review LVAD educational materials and track their individual data which has the potential to reduce readmissions [32–34].

Traditionally, the LVAD patient would remain associated with that implanting facility, regardless of the patient's distance traveled to the facility, socioeconomic limitations, time constraints and other factors. While this model encourages continuity of care in large cities with multiple healthcare centers, it discourages use of advanced therapies in patients who live outside of large cities [35, 36].

4. A new model: shared care

As the prevalence of end-stage heart disease continues to increase, the concept of "shared care" that focuses on implanting devices at a major institution and

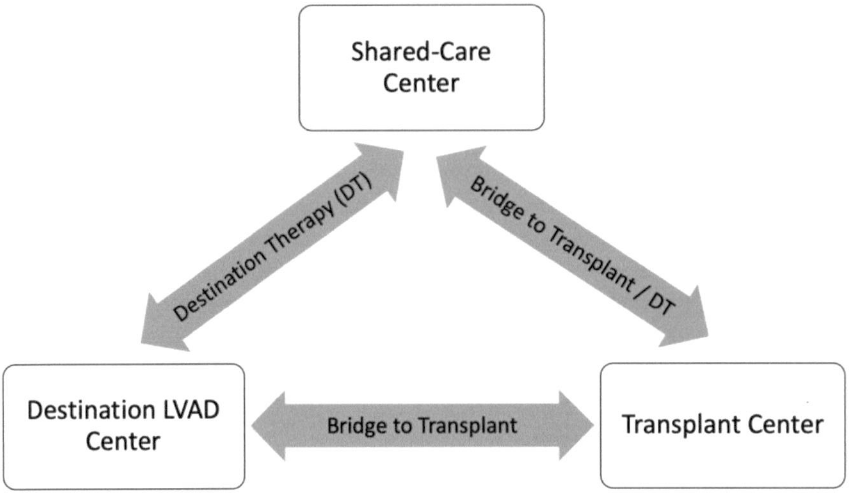

Figure 1.
Shared-care model for LVAD patients.

subsequently transferring follow up care to local heart failure cardiologists may expand access for LVADs to patients living in remote areas or of lower socioeconomic status who are unable to afford travel. In technical terms, a shared care LVAD center model occurs when a patient undergoes LVAD implantation at an implanting center, but greater than 50% of both the outpatient care and inpatient care alike is delivered locally [37]. This network of shared care sites can offload non-implant related issues from an implant center reducing strain on its resources while also allowing patients quicker access to routine care. In order for this to work, all care sites need to be properly trained in LVADs (**Figure 1**).

The shared-care model has been used among various specialties in medicine. In Toronto, it is being used in kidney transplant recipients with optimization of post-transplant care leading to a reduction in financial burden for patients and a reduction in follow up care volume for transplant centers [38]. They have also coordinated extensively in management of complex hematologic disorders which was initiated at Princess Margaret Cancer Centre. These models require training for community partners to ensure patient safety and satisfaction [39]. Later, it carried over to cardiology as the International Society of Heart and Lung Transplantation established guidelines for the principles of shared care after heart transplantation [40]. Now, it can be reiterated for the continuum of LVAD care.

While the model itself has been successfully implemented in complex medical conditions, it had not previously been attempted for LVAD patients. There are several examples demonstrating the success of the shared care model for LVAD patients. The Deborah Heart and Lung Center (DHLC) located in Browns Mills, New Jersey is a non-profit cardiac care specialty hospital which serves a largely underserved population in rural South Jersey. Its advanced heart failure program launched in April 2017 with partnerships and guidance from Thomas Jefferson University Hospitals, Temple University Hospital, and Robert Wood Johnson University Hospital. The shared care team consists of heart failure specialists and advanced practice providers [11]. Patients who lived in this area no longer had to travel over 90 minutes by car each way for their appointments nor did they require transfer to distant hospitals every time they were hospitalized. This allowed for all preop work-up and post-op care to occur in the local community, leading to improved access for patients with financial difficulties. This also improved patient compliance and diligence in attending all appointments, including seeking care as soon as issues arise. Other centers in the U.S. have demonstrated similar favorable outcomes with the shared-care model. A study published in JACC evaluated several key measures for LVAD patients implanted at the University of Utah Hospital. The authors included 336 patients implanted between 2007 and 2018, and categorized them based on level of care and resources utilized for their post implantation care. Overall, the rates of infection, bleeding, death, and pump thromboses were similar between care provided at the implanting institution (traditional care model) and outpatient care with LVAD specific training (the shared-care model). Rates were higher when outpatient services that were utilized did not have LVAD specific training, highlighting the importance of ensuring proper LVAD-specific training and resources are available at shared-care facilities [41].

There are no established criteria for shared care programs. However, a group of authors suggested several criteria that were published in the American Heart Association Journal Circulation, which focused on three broad categories: personnel, education, and equipment (**Table 1**). It is generally agreed that a shared care center should have an appointed local LVAD specialist—typically a heart failure cardiologist, though formal training in advanced heart failure is not a Joint Commission requirement for LVAD implantation facilities. Moreover, a nurse coordinator is another essential team member, who often serves as the primary contact for patients and other providers in the shared care team. Regarding education, LVAD specific training for all team members is essential. Preceptorships and LVAD vendors can provide the on-site education needed to learn the principles of LVAD management. Basic equipment should be garnered by the shared care facility and appropriate staff trained on its use. Device consoles, spare parts such as controllers, power cables, controller batteries, battery charges, and driveline equipment should ideally be available for timely replacement and troubleshooting [42].

Every follow-up visit starts with a review of systems concerning potential LVAD complications (**Table 2**). Next, is a blood pressure check which in continuous flow

General	• Dedicated LVAD Team
	• Physician Supervision—often a Cardiologist
	• Advanced Heart Failure Physician as Medical Director
	• Nurse Coordinator
	• Hotline or other dedicated LVAD patient portal
Education	• LVAD evaluation and management training
	• Implanting facility preceptorships
	• Internal review to continuously update best practices
	• Onsite LVAD training
	• VEndor sponsored, hands-on training
Maintenance	• Equipment: system monitors, batteries, controllers, driveline dressings
	• Establish policies for common complications
	• Interval reassessment of shared-care providers and patient outcomes

Table 1.
Potential criteria for shared-care partners.

Symptom	Evaluate for
Shortness of breath or leg swelling	Heart failure
Darkened or bloody urine or stools	Coagulation abnormalities—bleeding or pump thrombosis
Fevers, chills, or trauma to driveline site	Infection of driveline site

Table 2.
Symptoms in an LVAD patient.

devices is typically taken as a mean arterial pressure obtained via doppler. This is done by inflating the sphygmomanometer to 20 mmHg above flow occlusion and the opening pressure is considered the systolic blood pressure if the patient has pulsatility. In absence of pulsatility, as in most LVAD patients, this is considered the MAP or mean arterial pressure. Recommended MAP is 60–80 mmHg [43] and MAPs outside of this range warrant intervention. One of the common alarms is "low flow" due to decrease in pump flow in both hyper and hypotension. Guideline directed medical therapy or neurohormonal antagonism must be continued to appropriately control blood pressure.

An ECG is recommended in every LVAD patient to evaluate for ventricular arrhythmias. Prompt attention to any signs and symptoms of right heart failure should warrant further investigation. Alarm interrogation and documentation is also necessary. Critical alarms include "VAD stopped" and "critical battery" of 5 minutes which display as a red triangle. A yellow flashing triangle necessitates evaluation by a LVAD specialist as it suggests the pump exceeds its power threshold. Non-flashing alerts require non-emergent evaluation and can be evaluated at the shared care center.

Additionally, laboratory tests are followed closely to ensure proper function of the LVAD. Regular INR checks, lactate dehydrogenase (LDH), and plasma free hemoglobin or hematocrit are measured regularly to monitor for adequate anticoagulation, as well as to monitor for hemolysis [44]. In addition, echocardiography is used to monitor ventricular function. Aortic valve insufficiency symbolizes inadequate function and leads to adjustment to LVAD parameters [45].

Driveline exit sites must be thoroughly inspected and suspicion of infection should be followed up with site culture, blood cultures, and appropriate imaging studies. This can be performed at the local shared care site as it does not require hardware manipulation. As infection rates are higher in this population and linked to a higher 1-year mortality, prompt treatment of infections with appropriate antibiotics is warranted [46]. GI bleeding is another complication that needs prompt evaluation and can be completed at any shared care site with GI services. As arteriovenous malformations (AVMs) are frequently the source of GI bleeding, urgent endoscopy can serve as diagnostic and therapeutic modality [47]. Reversal of INR is not ideal and requires careful monitoring as subtherapeutic states lead to pump thrombosis and failure. Neurologic complications, both hemorrhagic and cardioembolic strokes account for 19% mortality following an LVAD implant [12]. Due to its increasing prevalence, guidelines for LVAD patients were added to the cardiopulmonary resuscitation (CPR) algorithm in 2017. All staff at shared care centers must be able to recognize situations in which this protocol must be initiated. If the device hum is present, then controller function and adequate power must be confirmed. In the absence of the device hum, with MAP <50 mmHg, CPR should be initiated. However, with increasing time of pump discontinuation, the likelihood of pump thrombosis increases.

Extracorporeal membrane oxygenation (ECMO) can be considered in these scenarios if CPR is successful and further care should be transferred to a tertiary center [48].

Follow up care in an LVAD patient is key to a successful outcome (**Figure 2**). Houston Methodist, another implanting center who successfully employs the shared care model, developed an extensive protocol to be used at shared care sites and specified the steps taken for equipment checks from patient education to clinician verification [49]. Educating the new shared care site on management of LVAD visits and emergencies can be a challenge. There are no current guidelines on the training required by ancillary staff to conduct such visits. Allowing for this care to occur near a patient's home can prove to be a psychosocial advantage, encouraging family members involvement and support. If a regional center is trained in the basics of LVAD management, it would decrease inpatient transfers for non-LVAD related hospitalizations, thereby improving patient experience while increasing community hospital revenue [50].

The success of the shared care model can also allow former non-implantation sites to naturally evolve into implantation sites themselves. The lessons learned by its participation as a shared care site enabled DHLC to develop its own LVAD transplant program further expanding patient access to needed durable mechanical support. New implant centers will then develop their own selection committee for candidacy in accordance with the International Society of Heart and Lung Transplant Committee standards and guidelines. The patient is scored on the

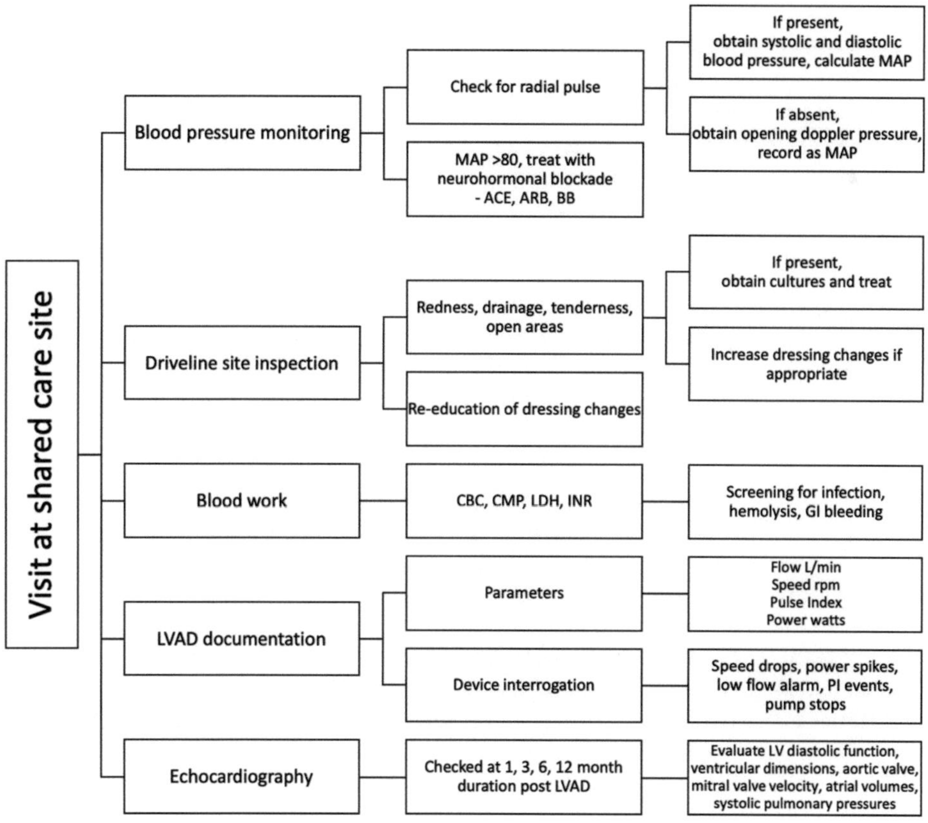

Figure 2.
Follow up evaluation of LVAD patient.

Interagency Registry for Mechanically Assisted Circulatory Support (INTERMACS) scale with 1 noting critical cardiogenic shock and 3 as stable on continuous intravenous inotropic support. INTERMACS 4 through 7 are not typically considered for LVAD as they have not yet reached the severity level required and are managed with medications. Once the case is reviewed by the team, patients with an INTERMACS score greater than two can choose the location for further work up for implantation with a plethora of tests such as echocardiograms, CT scans, and colonoscopies which are used to maximize the patient's status for an optimal outcome. Once a LVAD is implanted, follow up care is transferred back to the referring heart failure specialist who can continue to manage the patient in conjunction with the LVAD team. While heart transplantation remains the goal for some patients, others have been rejected due to age or other comorbidities. With the increasing demand for LVADs as destination therapy, more shared care networks will likely make the transition to implantation centers as well.

5. Discussion

The shared care to destination therapy model is an example of a new milestone in the advancement of care in the face of a growing heart failure pandemic. This model not only expands access to LVAD care, but also provides patients with social, financial, and satisfaction benefits. Shared care centers allow individuals to reach an advanced heart failure specialist quickly and efficiently by eliminating long distance travel and its associated financial expenses, as well as eliminating the excessive time commitment previously required for routine care. Patients are able to continue to reside in their own communities without making a lifelong commitment to either move where resources are available or spend an excessive amount of time traveling. The physician-to-patient ratios will remain lower enabling the physician-patient relationship to grow stronger over the years, which can improve the physician's ability to deliver personalized care and treat each patient based on their individual needs.

Given the high mortality rates in end stage heart failure and the recent advancements in LVAD technology that now afford a 3 year survival rate comparable to that of heart transplants [12], the demand for LVADs continues to escalate. Just as DHLC implemented the shared care to destination therapy model to eventually become a LVAD implant center, other shared care centers will likely do the same and heart failure cardiologists will be better able to evaluate adHF patients for LVAD candidacy to improve patient outcomes, satisfaction, and quality of life. This involves a multidisciplinary team discussing LVAD selection criteria, action plans, patient support, guideline directed treatment, and comprehensive follow up care.

A successful transition to a destination therapy center consists of a multidisciplinary team made up of an advanced heart failure cardiologist, LVAD surgical director, LVAD medical director, medical critical care director, heart failure nurse practitioners, and two social workers all centered on patient care. Through this period of expansion and development, these multidisciplinary teams are integral to the successful establishment of a shared care center and a LVAD implant center. As former shared care centers transition to destination therapy centers, the network of shared care can then expand outward even more.

DOI: http://dx.doi.org/10.5772/intechopen.111381

6. Limitations

A prospective study interrogating the shared-care model has yet to be performed. While limited data points are available, and retrospective data such as that from the centers mentioned above, the viewpoints in this chapter should be validated in a true prospective study. Such data will better delineate clinical outcomes for shared-care patients, such as adverse events, quality of life, financial impact for patients and healthcare systems. Despite a lack of such studies, the shared-care model is currently being utilized across the country.

7. Conclusion

Traditionally, because LVAD implant facilities are frequently remotely located from the patients that they serve, the shared-care model developed has demonstrated a safe and effective way to care for LVAD patients who live far from their implanting center.

Acknowledgements

The authors would like to acknowledge the contributions of Heart Failure and LVAD teams at DHLC, including but limited to Dr. Cindy Kos D.O., Abroo Muzaffar APN, Jamie McLeod, LPN, Dionne Bademosi APN, and Carlos Lozano APN.

Conflict of interest

The authors declare no conflict of interest.

Thanks

Special thanks to our colleagues, the Cardiovascular Disease Fellows at Deborah Heart and Lung Center.

Author details

Michael Sobieraj[1*], Antonio Valone[1], Brisha Bhikadiya[2], Ricardo Chia[1] and Kulpreet Barn[3]

1 Cardiovascular Disease Fellowship, Sidney Kimmel Medical College at Thomas Jefferson University Hospital/Deborah Heart and Lung Center, Browns Mills, NJ, USA

2 Internal Medicine Residency, Philadelphia College of Osteopathic Medicine, Philadelphia, PA, USA

3 Deborah Heart and Lung Center, Browns Mills, NJ, USA

*Address all correspondence to: sobierajm@deborah.org

References

[1] Chair SY, Yu DS, Ng MT, et al. Evolvement of left ventricular assist device: The implications on heart failure management. Journal of Geriatric Cardiology. 2016;**13**(5):425-430. DOI: 10.11909/j.issn.1671-5411.2016.05.015

[2] Severino P, Mather PJ, Pucci M, et al. Advanced heart failure and end-stage heart failure: Does a difference exist. Diagnostics (Basel). 2019;**9**(4):2170. DOI: 10.3390/diagnostics9040170

[3] Benjamin EJ, Blaha MJ, Chiuve SE, et al. Heart disease and stroke statistics-2017 update: A report from the American heart association. Circulation. 2017;**135**(10):e146-e603

[4] Young BA. Health disparities in advanced heart failure treatment: The intersection of race and sex. JAMA Network Open. 2020;**3**(7) e2011034. DOI: 10.1001/jamanetworkopen.2020.11034

[5] Gal TB et al. Guidance on the management of left ventricular assist device (LVAD) supported patients for the non-LVAD specialist healthcare provider: Executive summary. European Journal of Heart Failure. 2021;**23**:1597-1609

[6] Friedrich EB, Böhm M. Management of end stage heart failure. Heart. 2007;**93**(5):626-631. DOI: 10.1136/hrt.2006.098814

[7] Habal MV, Garan AR. Long-term management of end-stage heart failure. Best Practice & Research. Clinical Anaesthesiology. 2017;**31**(2):153-166. DOI: 10.1016/j.bpa.2017.07.003.Epub 2017 Jul 18

[8] Kalmanovich E, Audurier Y, Akodad M, Mourad M, Battistella P, Agullo A, et al. Management of advanced heart failure: A review. Expert Review of Cardiovascular Therapy. 2018;**16**((11):775-794. DOI: 10.1080/14779072.2018.1530112. Epub 2018 Oct 15

[9] Rose-Jones LJ. Heart failure: Advanced refractory heart failure. FP Essentials. Jul 2021;**506**:31-42

[10] Čerlinskaitė K, Javanainen T, Cinotti R, Mebazaa A. Global research on acute conditions team (GREAT) network. Acute heart failure management. Korean Circulation Journal. 2018;**48**(6):463-480. DOI: 10.4070/kcj.2018.0125

[11] Singhvi A, Trachtenberg B. Left ventricular assist devices 101: Shared Care for General Cardiologists and Primary Care. Journal of Clinical Medicine. 2019;**8**(10):1720. DOI: 10.3390/jcm8101720

[12] Kormos RL, Cowger J, Pagani FD, Teuteberg JJ, Goldstein DJ, Jacobs JP, et al. The Society of Thoracic Surgeons Intermacs database annual report: Evolving indications, outcomes, and scientific partnerships. The Journal of Heart and Lung Transplantation. 2019;**38**:114-126

[13] Goldstein DL, Meyns B, Xie R, Cowger J, Pettit S, Nakatani T, et al. Third annual report from the ISHLT mechanically assisted circulatory support registry: A comparison of centrifugal and axial continuous-flow left ventricular assist devices. The Journal of Heart and Lung Transplantation. 2019;**38**:352-363

[14] Mehra MR, Uriel N, Naka Y, et al. On behalf of the MOMENTUM 3 investigators. A fully magnetically levitated left ventricular assist device — Final

report. The New England Journal of Medicine. 2019;**380**:1618-1627

[15] Cowger JA, Stulak JM, Shah P, et al. Impact of center left ventricular assist device volume on outcomes after implantation: An INTERMACS analysis. JACC. Heart failure. 2017;**5**:691-699

[16] Wordingham SE, Mcllvennan CE. Palliative care for populations on mechanical circulatory support. AMA Journal of Ethics. 2019;**23**(5):E435-E442

[17] DeFiglio C, Lee A, Ashmont L, Dallas J. Treating the post-LVAD patient in an acute inpatient rehabilitation setting: An interdisciplinary approach to care and the roles of occupational, physical, and speech therapy. Rehab management: The interdisciplinary. Journal of Rehabilitation. 2021;**2021/2022**(Special Issue):20-27

[18] Eckman PM, John R. Bleeding and thrombosis in patients with continuous-flow ventricular assist devices. Circulation. 2012;**125**:3038-3047. DOI: 10.1161/CIRCULATIONAHA.111.040246

[19] Andreas M, Moayedifar R, Wieselthaler G, Wolzt M, Riebandt J, Haberl T, et al. Increased thromboembolic events with dabigatran compared with vitamin K antagonism in left ventricular assist device patients: A randomized controlled pilot trial. Circulation. Heart Failure. 2017;**10**(5):e003709. DOI: 10.1161/CIRCHEARTFAILURE.116.003709. PMID: 28500254; PMCID: PMC5434960

[20] Miller LW, Guglin M. Patient selection for ventricular assist devices: A moving target. Journal of the American College of Cardiology. 2013;**61**(12):1209-1221. DOI: 10.1016/j.jacc.2012.08.1029

[21] Yarboro LT, Bergin JD, Kennedy JL, Ballew CC, Benton EM, Ailawadi G, et al. Technique for minimizing and treating driveline infections. Annals of Cardiothoracic Surgery. 2014;**3**(6):557-562. DOI: 10.3978/j.issn.2225-319X.2014.09.08. PMID: 25512894; PMCID: PMC4250551

[22] Eckman PM, Dhungel V, Mandras S, Brisco MA, Emani S, Duval S, et al. Sexual function after left ventricular assist device. Journal of the American College of Cardiology. 2013;**61**:2021-2022

[23] Hanke JS, Riebandt J, Wahabzada M, Nur F, Wahabzada A, Dogan G, et al. Driving after left ventricular assist device implantation. Artificial Organs. 2018;**42**:695-699

[24] Cogswell R, Rafei AE, Cowger J, et al. Defining LVAD success: A nationwide survey of LVAD program team members. Journal of Heart and Lung Transplantation. 2020;**39**(4):S180-S181. DOI: 10.1016/j.healun.2020.01.760

[25] Giraldo-Grueso M, Webre K, Bansal A, Parrino P. Does patients with higher education have better postoperative results after LVAD implantation? Journal of Heart and Lung Transplantation. 2022;**41**(4):S162. DOI: 10.1016/j.healun.2022.01.381

[26] Foo JJ. Left ventricular assist device (LVAD) in Singapore: A Nation's 10 year experience. Journal of Heart and Lung Transplantation. 2020;**39**(4):S393. DOI: 10.1016/j.healun.2020.01.519

[27] Imamura T, Nguyen A, Rodgers D, Kim G, Raikhelkar J, Sarswat N, et al. Omega-3 therapy is associated with reduced gastrointestinal bleeding in patients with continuous-flow left ventricular assist device. Circulation. Heart Failure. 2018;**11**(10):e005082. DOI: 10.1161/CIRCHEARTFAILURE.118.005082. Erratum in: Circ Heart Fail. 2018 Nov;11(11):e000030

[28] Noriega BS, Sanchez-Gonzalez MA, Salyakina D, Coffman J. Understanding the impact of Omega-3 rich diet on the gut microbiota. Case Reports in Medicine. 2016;**2016**:3089303. DOI: 10.1155/2016/3089303

[29] Schlöglhofer T, Zapusek L, Wiedemann D, Riebandt J, Wittmann F, Dimitrov K, et al. International normalized ratio test frequency in left ventricular assist device patients affects anticoagulation quality and adverse events. ASAIO Journal. 2021;**67**(2):157-162. DOI: 10.1097/MAT.0000000000001206

[30] Stonebraker C, Lee A, Siddiqi U, et al. A model for continued LVAD patient success: A 4-year readmission-free HeartMate 3 postoperative course. Journal of Cardiac Surgery. 2021;**36**(3):1159-1161. DOI: 10.1111/jocs.15393

[31] Kuyumjian YM, Miyares MA, Leverock J, Chaparro S, Baker WL, Jennings DL. A multidisciplinary team-based process improves outpatient anticoagulation quality with continuous-flow left-ventricular assist devices. International Journal of Cardiology. 2016;**218**:118-119. DOI: 10.1016/j.ijcard.2016.05.030

[32] Luke A, Taveras M, Castillo C, et al. Early experience with a telehealth platform in LVAD patients. Journal of Heart and Lung Transplantation. 2020;**39**(4):S494. DOI: 10.1016/j.healun.2020.01.077

[33] Vidula H, Cheyne C, Martens J, Gosev I, Zareba W, Goldenberg I. Telehealth for the management of left ventricular assist device patients: The university of Rochester TeleLVAD Study. Journal of Cardiac Failure. 2021;**27**(1):112-113. DOI: 10.1016/j.cardfail.2020.10.001 Epub 2020 Oct 6

[34] Reiss N, Wegner KK, Hoffmann JD, Schulte Eistrup S, Boeken U, Morshuis M, et al. Requirements for a telemedicine center to monitor LVAD patients. Studies in Health Technology and Informatics. 2019;**260**:146-153

[35] Ibarra A, Howard-Quijano K, Hickey G, Garrard W, Thoma F, Mahajan A, et al. The impact of socioeconomic status in patients with left ventricular assist devices (LVADs). Journal of Cardiac Surgery. 2021;**36**(10):3501-3508. DOI: 10.1111/jocs.15794 Epub 2021 Jul 9

[36] Alonso WW, Faulkner KM, Pozehl BJ, Hupcey JE, Kitko LA, Lee CS. A longitudinal comparison of health-related quality of life in rural and urban recipients of left ventricular assist devices. Research in Nursing & Health. 2020;**43**(4):396-406. DOI: 10.1002/nur.22052 Epub 2020 Jul 6

[37] Shah M, Hafeez Y, Burns P, Toyoda Y, Moshiyakhov M, Neary M, et al. Shared care to destination therapy left ventricular assist device site: A novel strategy to start a successful mechanical circulatory support program. Current Cardiology Reports. 2021;**23**(8):112. DOI: 10.1007/s11886-021-01533-z

[38] Ashwin M, Minkovich M, Famure O, Kim SJ. Examining shared-care models for the long-term management of stable kidney transplant recipients. Transplantation. 2018;**102**(Suppl 7S-1):S537. DOI: 10.1097/01.tp.0000543385.82030.da

[39] Cheung V, Siddiq N, Devlin R, McNamara C, Gupta V. Shared-care model for complex chronic haematological malignancies. Canadian Oncology Nursing Journal. 2021;**31**(2):165-174. DOI: 10.5737/23688076312165174

[40] Costanzo MR, Dipchand A. International Society of Heart and Lung Transplantation Guidelines. The International Society of Heart and Lung Transplantation Guidelines for the care of heart transplant recipients. The Journal of Heart and Lung Transplantation. 2010;**29**:914-956. DOI: 10.1016/j.healun.2010.05.03

[41] Kiernan M, Joseph S. Sharing the care of mechanical circulatory support. Circulation: Heart Failure. 2015;**8**:629-635

[42] Yin M, Strege J, et al. Impact of shared care in remote areas for patients with left ventricular assist devices. JACC: Heart Failure. 2020;**8**(4):302-312

[43] Lanier GM, Orlanes K, Hayashi Y, Murphy J, Flannery M, Te-Frey R, et al. Validity and reliability of a novel slow cuff-deflation system for noninvasive blood pressure monitoring in patients with continuous-flow left ventricular assist device. Circulation. Heart Failure. 2013;**6**:1005-1012

[44] Shin DA, Lee JC, Shin H, Cho YJ, Kim HC. Point-of-care testing of plasma free hemoglobin and hematocrit for mechanical circulatory support. Scientific Reports. 15 Feb 2021;**11**(1):3788. DOI: 10.1038/s41598-021-83327-5

[45] Uriel N, Morrison KA, Garan AR, Kato TS, Yuzefpolskaya M, Latif F, et al. Development of a novel echocardiography ramp test for speed optimization and diagnosis of device thrombosis in continuous-flow left ventricular assist devices: The Columbia ramp study. Journal of the American College of Cardiology. 2012;**60**:1764-1775

[46] Gordon RJ, Weinberg AD, Pagani FD, Slaughter MS, Pappas PS, Naka Y, et al. Ventricular assist device infection study, prospective, multicenter study of ventricular assist device infections. Circulation. 2013;**127**:691-702

[47] Dakik HK, McGhan AA, Chiu ST, Patel CB, Milano CA, Rogers JG, et al. The diagnostic yield of repeated endoscopic evaluation in patients with gastrointestinal bleeding and left ventricular assist devices. Digestive Diseases and Sciences. 2016;**61**:1603-1610

[48] Peberdy MA, Gluck JA, Ornato JP, Bermudez CA, Griffin RE, Kasirajan V, et al. Cardiopulmonary resuscitation in adults and children with mechanical circulatory support: A scientific statement from the American Heart Association. Circulation. 2017;**135**:e1115-e1134

[49] Estep JD, Trachtenberg BH, Loza LP, Bruckner BA. Continuous flow left ventricular assist devices: Shared care goals of monitoring and treating patients. Methodist DeBakey Cardiovascular Journal. 2015;**11**(1):33-44. DOI: 10.14797/mdcj-11-1-33

[50] Kiernan MS, Joseph SM, Katz JN, et al. Sharing the care of mechanical circulatory support: Collaborative efforts of patients/caregivers, shared-care sites, and left ventricular assist device implanting centers. Circulation. Heart Failure. 2015;**8**(3):629-635. DOI: 10.1161/CIRCHEARTFAILURE.114.001767